Psychoanalytic Thinking in Occupational Therapy

T0261209

Psychoanalytic Thinking in Occupational Therapy
Symbolic, Relational and Transformative

Dr Lindsey Nicholls
School of Health Science and Social Care
Brunel University, London, UK

Julie Cunningham Piergrossi
The Vivaio Centre: Practice, Training and Research in Psychoanalytic
Occupational Therapy
University of Milan, Milan, Italy

Carolina de Sena Gibertoni
The Vivaio Centre: Practice, Training and Research in Psychoanalytic
Occupational Therapy
University of Milan, Milan, Italy

Margaret A. Daniel
Clinical Specialist Occupational Therapist in Psychotherapy
Lansdowne Psychotherapy Service, Glasgow, UK

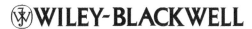
WILEY-BLACKWELL

A John Wiley & Sons, Ltd., Publication

This edition first published 2013
© 2013 by John Wiley & Sons, Ltd

Wiley-Blackwell is an imprint of John Wiley & Sons, formed by the merger of Wiley's global Scientific, Technical and Medical business with Blackwell Publishing.

Registered office: John Wiley & Sons, Ltd, The Atrium, Southern Gate, Chichester, West Sussex, PO19 8SQ, UK

Editorial offices: 9600 Garsington Road, Oxford, OX4 2DQ, UK
The Atrium, Southern Gate, Chichester, West Sussex, PO19 8SQ, UK
2121 State Avenue, Ames, Iowa 50014-8300, USA

For details of our global editorial offices, for customer services and for information about how to apply for permission to reuse the copyright material in this book please see our website at www.wiley.com/wiley-blackwell.

The right of the author to be identified as the author of this work has been asserted in accordance with the UK Copyright, Designs and Patents Act 1988.

All rights reserved. No part of this publication may be reproduced, stored in a retrieval system, or transmitted, in any form or by any means, electronic, mechanical, photocopying, recording or otherwise, except as permitted by the UK Copyright, Designs and Patents Act 1988, without the prior permission of the publisher.

Designations used by companies to distinguish their products are often claimed as trademarks. All brand names and product names used in this book are trade names, service marks, trademarks or registered trademarks of their respective owners. The publisher is not associated with any product or vendor mentioned in this book. This publication is designed to provide accurate and authoritative information in regard to the subject matter covered. It is sold on the understanding that the publisher is not engaged in rendering professional services. If professional advice or other expert assistance is required, the services of a competent professional should be sought.

Library of Congress Cataloging-in-Publication Data
Psychoanalytic thinking in occupational therapy : symbolic, relational, and transformative / Lindsey Nicholls . . . [et al.].
      p. ; cm.
  Includes bibliographical references and index.
  ISBN 978-0-470-65586-3 (pbk. :alk. paper)
  I. Nicholls, Lindsey.
  [DNLM: 1.   Occupational Therapy–psychology. 2.   Psychoanalytic Theory. 3.   Psychotherapy. WM 450.5.O2]
  616.89′165–dc23
                                                                                      2012027805

A catalogue record for this book is available from the British Library.

Wiley also publishes its books in a variety of electronic formats. Some content that appears in print may not be available in electronic books.

Cover images: © iStockphoto/tuja66
Cover design by Sandra Heath

Set in 10/12 pt Sabon by Thomson Digital, Noida, India

1   2013

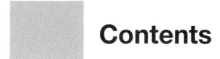

Contents

Foreword

From the day that I first learned about the work of Azima and Azima (1959) and Fidler and Fidler (1963) whilst undertaking my occupational therapy course in the mid to late 1960s in Glasgow, I was captivated. This work sought to explore and understand the meaning of what we do as human beings and how participation in occupational therapy could offer another means of communication. The Fidlers also contributed one of the first and most comprehensive approaches to activity analysis. I was fascinated by the links between psychoanalytic thinking and the practice of occupational therapy and was lucky enough in my early practice to work in a unit which was underpinned by the principles of group psychotherapy and the importance of the milieu. Forty-five years later, I am equally engrossed by the ideas offered in this text.

Over the years, I have reflected countless times on how the ideas, concepts and principles have informed my understanding and work, whether that was in practice, education, management or research. Historically, there has always been a sustained adherence to this way of understanding human beings within the occupational literature. Contrary to the popular view of some occupational therapy theorists who considered that therapists who thought and practised in this way would lead to the demise of the profession, I maintain that this form of thinking enhances our repertoire of knowledge and skill. I endorse the view that is taken in this book that occupation is symbolic, relational and transformative, and to facilitate understanding of this we need to refer to the seminal work referred to in this text.

This is a courageous book. It bravely runs counter to contemporary discourse of health and social care and reminds us of what it is to be a therapist by attending to multi-layered communication and containing distress. Therapy is characterised by providing emotional safety and containment. Often engagement with occupation provides that safe space to begin to explore difficult issues. Throughout, the book strives to help the reader develop their own sensitivity to others through the provision of vignettes and this both helps deepen professional reasoning and links theory with practice. This is the crux of good educational practice and enables readers to risk reflecting upon and considering their own interactions with others. It is also courageous in adhering to the principles and mores of psychoanalytical thinking instead of the more popular notion in occupational therapy literature of psychodynamic thinking.

The writers have outlined the links between psychoanalytical thought and the practice of occupational therapy in a developmental way by revisiting seminal works from both occupational therapy and psychoanalysis. Additionally, they have offered a specific model to infuse practice with a celebration of the therapeutic use of self and the pivotal contribution of emotion and relationships in the lives of human beings. The text covers work from childhood to later adulthood and reveals how this way of working with people can facilitate the development of an emotional language and enable emotional shifts to occur. It also covers how work of this nature can revitalise supervision and develop organisations in a positive way. The final chapters of this text concern psychoanalytic thinking in research and this reveals how there has been a regeneration of interest in the contribution of psychoanalytical thinking within social science. As such the book unites theory, practice and research.

I have found this a refreshing text with the authoritative signature of stimulating the occupational imagination to creatively work with the unconscious. It encourages practitioners to strive to understand internal life, whether as a therapist, educator, researcher or manager. While it may only be possible for a small number of occupational therapists to directly practise in this way, what this book offers is a way to enhance professional reasoning, deepen understanding of the meaning of occupation and contribute to mental health and well-being.

Dr Sheena E. E. Blair
Dip COT, M Ed, Ed D, FHEA, FCOT

Foreword

In the UK today we are experiencing a crisis in the quality of our care services with scandal after scandal surfacing in our hospitals, our residential homes and day services. In Europe, for two decades now, welfare services have struggled to develop under successive waves of management reforms which, under the banner 'getting more for less', have sought to increase the productivity of the public services. I think it is clear now that whilst in some cases we may have increased the volume of throughput, it has been largely achieved by a real decline in the quality of care. The danger is that as the OECD economies seek to regenerate private affluence on the backs of public austerity, the quality of care is something that will be seen as something we can no longer afford.

The appearance of *Psychoanalytic Thinking in Occupational Therapy* is therefore very timely. For here is a book which has the courage to proclaim that quality counts and that ultimately the only guarantee of quality lies in the richness of the relationship that emerges between the professional and the client. I deliberately use the unfashionable word 'client' rather than 'service user' because the latter has become a degraded term, a piece of 'carewash' (like greenwash) which actually covers up the lack of care which now seems to accompany the bizarre mish-mash of centralised control, micro-management and breakdown of real accountability which makes up our increasingly fragmented welfare system. The concept of 'client' (still used by architects, solicitors and many other professions) has those connotations of dignity, respect and status that we urgently need to rediscover to challenge the lack of care presently taking place.

Psychoanalytic Thinking in Occupational Therapy is unashamedly humanistic. It puts the humanity of the client at the forefront of the professional agenda – their emotions, frailties, eccentricities, strengths and mysteries. Indeed it pours out of the many vignettes and case studies that are such a marvellous feature of this book. Whilst the authors show great confidence in their use of psychoanalytic terms, they do so in a way which illuminates rather than reduces the humanity of their clients. This is how the psychoanalysis I love should be used – to enliven, to 'move' and to make you think, the opposite of jargon or dogma.

In contrast to the regimented, risk-averse and prescriptive techniques which have come to dominate our thinking about professional practice, the authors of this book offer an entirely different way forward. Can we afford *not* to move in the direction they point to? So much of our accounting these days is preoccupied with short-term efficiencies that the long-term costs of failing to think systemically pile up all around us. There are signs all about us that the citizen is no longer prepared to surrender public welfare on the altar of economic austerity. We do indeed deserve more. The kind of practices outlined in this book should lie at the heart of a welfare society, one which values human and non-human relations as intrinsic goods rather than means to an end.

Professor Paul Hoggett
Centre for Psycho-Social Studies, University of West England

Acknowledgements

We would like to thank our clients, colleagues and students for their sincerity, patience and commitment to work that can only truly be done in the spirit of collaborative inquiry.

1 Introduction

Lindsey Nicholls, Julie Cunningham Piergrossi,
Margaret Daniel and Carolina de Sena Gibertoni

There is a saying for people who plan to undertake the long-distance walking route known as the 'Way of St James': it states that the *Camino de Santiago*[1] begins when you first think of it. That is how the book began; we began to think of it. Since 2006 we have exchanged our thoughts in emails and initial writings, and used a process of peer editing to learn from each other and produce this book. We have found ways to meet in person and listen to each other's presentations (at Brunel University Master Class events and international conferences in 2009, 2010 and 2011), and this had led to our connecting with many other occupational therapists who have been using (i.e. thinking and working with) psychoanalysis as a theory and method within their clinical practice.

It has been a rich and rewarding time where each of the authors, at different times and/or in relation to certain specialist topics, has taken the lead. Although we come from diverse professional and personal backgrounds, we share a conviction in the importance of using psychoanalytic theory in occupational therapy. In this we have been good companions and learnt much from each other's clinical work and theoretical discussions. This book is a result of our collaborative desire to make this work available to scholars and clinical therapists, to form a wider 'community of practice' (Wenger, 1998), where new projects, clinical discussions and writing can emerge.

At its heart the book discusses the work that we have practised, learnt, thought about and carry within as we engage with clients, students and colleagues. Our hope is that the book will provide a basis for serious study by therapists who are interested in psychoanalytic theory and may have begun their own journey into the internal landscape of the emotional understanding of people and what they 'do'.

---

[1] The 1000-year-old pilgrimage to the shrine of St James in the Cathedral of Santiago de Compostela is known in English as the 'Way of St James' and in Spanish as the *Camino de Santiago*. Over 100,000 pilgrims travel to the city each year from points all over Europe and other parts of the world (Wikipedia, 2012).

Psychoanalytic Thinking in Occupational Therapy: Symbolic, Relational and Transformative, First Edition.
Lindsey Nicholls, Julie Cunningham Piergrossi, Carolina de Sena Gibertoni and Margaret A. Daniel.
© 2013 John Wiley & Sons, Ltd. Published 2013 by John Wiley & Sons, Ltd.

There are 13 chapters in all (including this one) and the book has been divided into three overarching themes; theory, application and research. The first section takes the classic psychoanalytic theories (e.g. Freud, Klein, Bion, Winnicott and Bowlby) and considers their influence on occupational therapy practice and thinking. The second section is devoted to an explanation of a psychoanalytic occupational therapy model (MOVI) and this is followed with further discussions of psychoanalysis in clinical occupational therapy practice. The final section describes research methods and projects that have incorporated psychoanalytic thinking in occupational therapy.

Each chapter could be read as an extended case study but we hope there is sufficient cross-reference between the different contributions to make for a coherent whole. In many ways it has been hard to choose the order of work for the linear structure that the book offered. The core of the book lies in understanding MOVI (Chapter 7), an occupational therapy model, and we would suggest that readers develop a duel vision where MOVI can be held in mind as they refer to the earlier chapters on Freud, Klein and Bion (Chapter 3), Bowlby (Chapter 5) and the therapeutic use of self (Chapter 2).

There are certain terms in current occupational therapy literature which have gained professional ascendance – for example, using the term 'client' rather than 'patient', and 'occupation' not 'activity' – which we have decided to use interchangeably. This is not a form of political rebellion against the discussions on client-centred practice or the value of understanding occupation, but belongs to the eclectic theoretical background we have used to develop an integration of psychoanalytic thinking in occupational therapy.

We are very grateful for the encouragement that Katrina Hulme-Cross, Rupert Cousens and Sara Crowley-Vigneau, the health sciences commissioning editors at Wiley-Blackwell, have given us during this time. Without their active support we might still have been thinking about writing the book and not have completed it!

Finding our way

In this section, each author introduces themselves to the reader, saying how it was that they began establishing a link between psychoanalysis and occupational therapy. We hope these brief introductions will provide an illustration of our individual (even idiosyncratic) and shared interests in using psychoanalytic thinking in our work as occupational therapists.

Lindsey Nicholls

In 2002, after my rather clumsy presentation at a mental health conference on the use of dreams in clinical work, I was generously invited by Jennifer Creek to contribute a chapter on my work for her forthcoming book, *Contemporary Issues in Occupational Therapy* (Creek and Lawson-Porter, 2007). It was a professional lifeline for me as I had recently moved to the UK from South Africa and found myself floundering in a discourse full of positive affirmations and seemingly (only) conscious intensions. Any consideration of the unconscious aspects of clients and professionals had been subsumed by an emphasis on partnership working and recovery. I attempted to give voice to my concerns about this loss of thoughtfulness about the unconscious:

> I have had an interest in and involvement with a psycho-analytic view of occupational therapy for so much of my professional life that I can no longer see clearly without these conceptual lenses.[2] It has been a concern to me that over the past 40 years a psychoanalytic discourse in occupational therapy has almost completely disappeared from our professional literature, except for a few voices (Banks and Blair, 1997; Cole, 1998; Collins, 2004; Daniel and Blair, 2002a; 2002b; Creek, 1997; Hagedorn, 1992), and it has been my wish to persuade occupational therapists to consider (or reconsider) what psychoanalysis can offer us in our endeavour to alleviate the suffering of our clients and support their sense of purpose in day to day life.
>
> (Nicholls, 2007, p. 58)

When I wrote this entreaty to the profession, much admiring and quoting Margaret Daniel's work, I didn't know we would meet, that she worked as a clinical specialist psychodynamic occupational therapist in Glasgow and that we would become friends. I didn't known that Julie Cunningham Piergrossi and Carolina de Sena Gibertoni were working in Milan, Italy, using an 'occupational play space' in which children and adolescents could discover aspects of themselves through their choice of objects and activity in the containing presence of a psychoanalytic occupational therapist.

Then a wonderful synchronistic event took place. In 2006 I was the first speaker in a group of four papers at the World Federation of Occupational Therapy (WFOT) in Sydney, Australia. My paper used the layered story from the book *Life of Pi* (Martel, 2003) as an illustration of the concerns I had with some of the concepts in 'client-centred practice': that it can ignore unconscious motives, ambivalent emotions and contradictory behaviour (see Chapter 2). The paper seemed to go well and when I sat down a woman moved to the seat next to me, clasped my wrist and asked me where I was going. I was a little alarmed at the strength of her grip and told her I would be staying until the end of the session. 'Good,' she said. 'I

---

[2] The idea of theory (structure) being used as a lens through which to view the world – 'a pair of spectacles with a specially tinted filter' – comes from Hagedorn (1992, p. 14).

didn't want you to disappear.' It was Julie and she gave the last talk in the group of four papers.

Julie's presentation described the response postgraduate students had to learning about the MOVI model (see Chapter 11). MOVI incorporates an understanding of the conscious and unconscious choices, actions and words of patients within the containing environment of a 'play space'; a room full of activity choices and a therapist. While hearing about their work in Italy, delivered in Julie's eloquent, measured voice, I began to cry. This work took into account the conscious and unconscious aspects of the client and therapist, through the communication involved in 'doing' something together. MOVI captured a way of thinking and working that was an alternative to the highly contested ground taken by other practice models (e.g. the MOHO, KAWA and CMOP). But in truth, my tearful response to her talk was because I no longer felt alone.

It was through Julie that I met her colleague and collaborator, the Italian author Carolina de Sena Gibertoni, and this completed the initial learning group. Carolina's knowledge and application of core psychoanalytic theory in occupational therapy has been important in locating the book in the classic psychoanalytic texts. I have valued what each author has contributed in their understanding of theory as lived through the experience of working with clients and activities in the intimate relational space of emotions.

Perhaps I can end my introduction with where I began: by paying attention to the unconscious. It has been in my personal analysis that I have found an inner coherence and capacity for creativity. My experience of psychoanalytic psychotherapy has given me a deep belief in the efficacy of this approach to working with others.

> I have never doubted the existence of the unconscious; in fact it was quite a relief when I realised during my first experience of an analysis, at the age of 23, that my dreams, thoughts and feelings were a language that I had not yet learnt to understand, but that were available to me as a guide to my internal life. Perhaps it is this investment in one's own internal life that is the most daunting and fulfilling in working within a psychoanalytic framework with clients. Bion (1991), an analyst who is considered a prodigious and original thinker, wrote in his autobiography that having recognised his most primitive self, capable of almost any heinous crime, he could better understand his clients and their struggles.
>
> (Nicholls, 2010, p. 32)

Julie Cunningham Piergrossi

The event that started out the adventure of this book for me was my meeting up with Lindsey Nicholls (already described by her) in 2006 at the World Congress in Sydney. By pure chance we were presenting our papers in the same session and she spoke before I did. I remember listening to her psychoanalytic discourse and being both astounded and delighted at how it fitted together with my own thoughts. At the same time she was opening my mind to new ideas and I remember running up to her immediately afterwards and asking her not to leave until I had spoken, that I needed to talk to her. I was afraid she would be lost in the more than 2000 therapists present and that I would never find her again. In the general discussion following my talk she asked me two pertinent and thought-provoking questions which are always such a gift in a situation like that. Later we began to talk together and we haven't stopped since.

My interest in psychoanalysis began when I studied occupational therapy in the USA back in the 1960s and has never wavered since, even though my profession has changed immensely in the intervening years.

When I arrived in Italy in 1969 I became part of a group of psychoanalysts called 'Il Ruolo Terapeutico', with whom I began my training which is still ongoing. My case presentations, in supervision together with colleagues who are psychoanalysts, have always aroused curiosity in some and consternation in others. It was difficult when I heard people I respected tell me that the presence of the activities and the materials during the therapy sessions could be an impediment to the therapeutic process. In 40 years of working together things have changed as I have learned to put words to my 'doing' and my colleagues have accepted the fact that baking a cake can have psychoanalytic potential.

'Ruolo Terapeutico' was instrumental in making clear for me the importance of the structure of the therapy as a container for the process, a concept which led to the understanding of choice as part of the setting (the structure) of the occupational therapy experience using the Vivaio Model (MOVI).

I am especially grateful to Sandro Bonomo for his continual support of my work. It was Sandro who helped me to really understand the emotions around choices, especially concerning the complex aspects of unpredictability and its therapeutic value. My psychotherapist colleague, Elisabeth de Verdiere, was another strong supporter of occupational therapy with a psychoanalytic theory base and helped Carolina and myself in the founding of 'Il Vivaio' and in developing and carrying out the training programme for MOVI. The constant exchange with Carolina during the development of our model is a natural part of my existence, and much of my learning has come from her. Supervision, written contributions to a professional psychoanalytic journal, reading groups, seminars and my own personal psychoanalysis have helped me on my way, and of course my best teachers have always been the children and their families who came to me for help.

I can never think about myself as psychoanalytically trained without thinking first about myself as an occupational therapist. I think I have been an occupational therapist from when I was a child playing with my grandmother's box of odds and ends. I have always loved 'doing': cooking, sewing, woodworking and just making and fixing things. Being able to use 'doing' (which has always been therapeutic for myself) for helping others has been a privilege and a huge stroke of luck in enabling me to have a job I love. Because occupational therapy did not exist when I arrived in Italy, part of my time has always been dedicated to developing and teaching the basic profession. I have always strongly stressed the importance of keeping occupations in occupational therapy.

As an American living and working in Italy I have had the privilege of knowing two cultures well. The Italian influence on my life and work has been enormous, and living in a country with people so relational and expressive of complex emotion has contributed to my understanding of that part of myself which in turn has helped me in my work with very sick children. At the same time, my American part was always encouraged by Carolina, who never tired of pointing out to me the positive aspects of my first and formative culture and how important it was to combine the two.

This book is a continuation of my 'conversations' with Lindsey and my exchanges with Carolina in an ongoing search for ways to further develop and implement clinical excellence in psychoanalytically oriented occupational therapy.

Margaret Daniel

I remember being interviewed to become a member of the Scottish Institute of Human Relations in Scotland and being asked how I knew that I had an unconscious. This thought still stays with me as a question that I only manage to glimpse at in myself, but can see much more easily in someone else, through slips of the tongue, forgotten agreements or an off-the-cuff remark. I am curious to know more about how our unconscious influences us, something we cannot see or be aware of in ourselves, yet which has such an impact on our experiences and choices, professionally, organisationally and socially.

My journey has been mainly based in Glasgow, where I am a Clinical Specialist Occupational Therapist in Psychotherapy. I have worked for over 35 years in the NHS where my career has been devoted to Mental Health and especially to the field of psychotherapy. I built up further training at the Scottish Institute of Human Relations and I have attained senior accreditation as a psychodynamic counsellor with the British Association of Counselling and Psychotherapy (BACP). I went on to gain a Master's degree in Psychoanalytic Studies from the University of Sheffield, in which I attempted to unite the dialogue between psychodynamic thinking and occupational therapy. In expanding my unique post as a clinical specialist I needed to find a way to identify and meet with other likeminded occupational therapists. This was limited in Scotland and an opportunity came about to develop a website called the National Exchange for Psychodynamic Occupational Therapists (NEPOT), which is a self-regulating intranet community that is located within the NHS Mental Health Specialist Library and aims to link and provide support for occupational therapists interested in psychodynamic thinking.

As a Member of the Scottish Institute of Human Relations I have been involved in the training of psychodynamic counsellors and worked in organisational consultancy projects which took psychodynamic thinking out into the voluntary and public sectors. It is in keeping with its founder, Jock Sutherland's philosophy of taking psychodynamic thinking beyond therapy and into the community. I was invited to become a Trustee of the Sutherland Trust, which carries on Sutherland's ideas by supporting human relations work in health, education and social services through the application of psychodynamic ideas and practices. One of the lectures introduced me to Dr Una McCluskey and her research work on adult attachment. I decided to join one of her groups for professional caregivers and have gone on to do further training in York in this approach and theory, which she developed in collaboration with Dorothy Heard and Brian Lake (Heard, Lake and McCluskey, 2009; Heard, McCluskey and Lake, 2011). For occupational therapists I believe this approach endorses how creative activities can validate and restore a person's sense of well-being. It also links with my work and interest in supervision, where a collaborative approach can enhance learning.

My connections to the other authors came through a chance meeting with the then Director of Occupational Therapy at Brunel University, Christine Craik, who was my first Head Occupational Therapist. She drew my attention to an article she thought might interest me, recently published by her colleague. I read Lindsey's article (Nicholls, 2003) and excitedly made contact as I had discovered someone else who was writing about the influence of the felt experience. This too was how I had felt on reading Julie and Carolina's work (Piergrossi and Gibertoni, 1999) while studying for my Master's. The chance of meeting and working with them was an incredible opportunity that I would never have imagined possible and has led to a cross-fertilising of ideas and interests.

I am ever indebted to the patience and generous feedback I received from my colleagues in occupation therapy, nursing, counselling and psychotherapy. I am also appreciative of the time that people took in reading over the material and helping me to fine tune my thoughts. Special thanks go to Samantha Flower, Sheena Blair, Sue Jervis, Eileen MacAlister, Una McCluskey and Paul Arnesen. I also need to thank my son, Kenny, for his support and endurance throughout this task.

Carolina de Sena Gibertoni

It was 1980 and I was visiting an Italian friend in London. We were having breakfast when her telephone rang and surprisingly it was for me. Who could be calling me in London? It was Gianna Polacco from the Tavistock Clinic, to whom I had written some time back, and she was arranging an appointment with Lina Generali Clements for an admissions interview for the Tavistock training programme in Milan. This was the moment that began my tie to the institution which illuminated my path of knowledge and contributed to transferring psychoanalytic concepts to our profession (occupational therapy).

I was working in Milan together with Julie Cunningham (who had come to Italy from America) and Elisabeth de Verdiere, a psychoanalytic psychotherapist working with severely disturbed autistic and psychotic children and adolescents. Julie had introduced me to occupational therapy using a model based on Gail Fidler's work. I became aware of areas of shadow, obscure aspects of what we were doing, curiosities that seemed to demand responses.

I had completed my own personal analysis and knowing myself better helped me to establish a different kind of relationship with my young patients and with their parents; it was as if their emotions and mine were entering and demanding space in the setting. I was continuing my training with Donata Miglietta e Mirella Curi Novelli in analytic psychodrama, and participating in psychoanalytic study groups with Corrao, Gaburri, Napolitani and the Roman group connected with the journal *Quaderni di Psicoterapia Infantile*. The Italian world of psychoanalysis was very lively. However, child psychoanalysis in Italy was just beginning. It was an experience that came from afar, particularly from the British world, and I felt the need to know more about children, to begin a training course like that proposed by the Tavistock Clinic. The appointment with Lina Clements had great importance for me, but how would the admission interview go?

It was a foggy Milanese afternoon and I remember the surprise when the door was opened by an elderly lady with a kind smile. She had me sit down and guided me easily into a conversation. After about an hour she told me I was suitable and could present a request for admission either to the course which would be starting in Milan two years later or to the one in Rome, where all of the teachers would be coming from the London Tavistock Clinic, which would begin that same year. I did not hesitate: if my application was accepted, I would choose Rome.

And that is how it all turned out. It was not easy for me. I was working; I had a family with two young children; the trip to Rome from Milan was long and costly; and there was an enormous amount of studying and preparation between one meeting and the next. But it was worth it! I presented my weekly 'Baby Observations' to Marta Harris and Donald Meltzer, and what I learned was often a surprise for me. Their seeming disagreements, fresh and lively, revealed two different points of view, full of wisdom in respect to how much movement could be seen in the observer, the baby and the whole context. As meeting after meeting passed in Baby Observations, learning to observe, paying attention to detail, finding an emotional resonance, became the instruments that would accompany me in my whole working life.

I took part in the Tavistock training for many years, attending seminars with Francis Tustin, Jeanne Magagna, Gianna Polacco, Menzies Lyth and Anton Obholzer in a precise training for working with groups. The Tavistock training, together with the Italian contributions, permitted me that 'fertile contamination' with occupational therapy which, up until then, was still confined to the goal of functional independence. I felt that it was time to release our occupational therapy from its medical constraints by giving it the new role of contemplating the dynamics of relationships that are born during clinical practice.

The rest is written in this book. For long decades Julie and I have worked side by side, exchanging ideas and presenting at national and international congresses. We have had continuous interaction with Italian colleagues, psychoanalysts and students both within and outside of the university in therapy rooms and in various institutions. The emotions that were discovered in our occupational therapy practice found a specific theoretical location when a relational model of occupational therapy (MOVI) was born.

> In recent years, following the happy coincidence of their meeting that Lindsey and Julie recount, we have participated in the Brunel Master Classes on Psychoanalytic Thinking in Occupational Therapy (2009, 2010, 2011). This has been an enriching experience, an exchange of thoughts with a common base that the far-sightedness of Lindsey willed into a book. And I stop here.
>
> If I think about it, the English and American influence on my working life was fundamental. And yet . . . I still cannot speak English with the same fluid thoughts that my mind has allowed.

Finding the words

As we have said earlier, this book was written to begin a conversation with our colleagues. Since 2006, when the four of us established a correspondence, we have had many contributions from – and lively discussions with – clinical and academic therapists, at the Brunel master classes and international conferences. Our book offers an opportunity to engage with the thinking and clinical work undertaken by occupational therapists who engage with the relational and symbolic world of the client. The case examples, embedded in every chapter, pay careful attention to the emotionally nuanced events that take place within and between therapist and client, and what is done (or not done) in the therapeutic encounter. It is within this relationship that a shift or change can take place in the inner world of the client. This is essentially slow, painstaking work where small emotional gains can be measured in the patient's capacity for creative thought and/or play. It is deeply rewarding work and, because therapists need to understand the conscious and unconscious experiences of the client, it is helpful for the therapist to have their own psychodynamic psychotherapy and supervision.

Conclusions

Once begun, the work of analysis through acknowledging feelings, thoughts, associations and reflections never ends. This work is the essence of relationships (love) and creativity (art, poetry and music). Freud stated that that wherever his theory led him, he found a poet had already been there. T. S. Eliot (1959) captures the struggle to articulate what is known, learnt from experience, better than any theoretical paper on the subject. As Palmer (1979) stated, using Eliot's work from East Coker, 'Trying to learn to use words, and every attempt . . . Is a wholly new start, and a different kind of failure' (p. 171). This quote seems to describe how difficult it is to articulate (find the words for) the discoveries of what it is to be human. This knowledge seems to be in a state of being found and lost, only to be found again. We are hoping that psychoanalytic thinking, which was present in the early theoretical papers on occupational therapy (Fidler and Fidler, 1963), will be found and enjoyed again by a wide collection of therapists.

References

Banks, E. J., and Blair, S. E. E. (1997) The contribution of occupational therapy within the context of the psychodynamic approach for older clients who have mental health problems. *Health Care in Later Life*, 2 (2), 85–92.

Cole, M. (1998) *Group Dynamics in Occupational Therapy*. Thorofare, NJ: Slack.

Collins, M. (2004) Dreaming and occupation. *British Journal of Occupational Therapy*, 67 (2), 96–98.

Creek, J. (1997) *Occupational Therapy in Mental Health* (2nd edn). London: Churchill Livingstone.

Creek, J. and Lawson-Porter, A. (eds) (2007) *Contemporary Issues in Occupational Therapy: Reasoning and Reflection*. Chichester: John Wiley & Sons, org.

Cunningham Piergrossi, J., and Gilbertoni, C. de Sena (1999) The importance of inner transformation in the activity process. *Occupational Therapy International*, 2, 36–47.

Daniel, M. A., and Blair, S. E. E. (2002a) A psychodynamic approach to clinical supervision: 1. *British Journal of Therapy and Rehabilitation*, 9 (6), 237–240.

Daniel, M. A., and Blair, S. E. E. (2002b) A psychodynamic approach to clinical supervision: 2. *British Journal of Therapy and Rehabilitation*, 9 (7), 274–277.

Eliot, T. S. (1959) *Four Quartets*. London: Faber.

Fidler, G., and Fidler, J. (1963) *Occupational Therapy as a Communication Process in Psychiatry*. New York: Macmillan.

Hagedorn, R. (1992) *Occupational Therapy: Foundations for Practice*. Edinburgh: Churchill Livingstone.

Heard, D., Lake, B., and McCluskey, U. (2009) *Attachment Therapy with Adolescents and Adults*. London: Karnac.

Heard, D., McCluskey, U., and Lake, B. (2011) *Attachment Therapy with Adolescents and Adults* (2nd edn). London: Karnac.

Martel, Y. (2003) *Life of Pi*. Edinburgh: Canongate.

Nicholls, L. (2003) Occupational therapy on the couch. *Therapy Weekly*, 10 July, 30 (2), 5.

Nicholls, L. (2007) A psychoanalytic discourse in occupational therapy. In J. Creek and A. Lawson-Porter (eds), *Contemporary Issues in Occupational Therapy: Reasoning and Reflection* (pp. 55–85). Chichester: John Wiley & Sons, org.

Nicholls, L. (2010) 'Putting it into words': A psychoanalytically orientated ethnographic study of hospital based clinical occupational therapy departments in the UK and South Africa. Unpublished PhD thesis, University of the West England, Bristol.

Palmer, B. (1979) Learning and the group experience. In W. G. Lawrence (ed.), *Exploring Individual and Organizational Boundaries* (pp. 169–192). London: Karnac.

Wenger, E. (1998) *Communities of Practice: Learning, Meaning, and Identity*. Cambridge: Cambridge University Press.

Wikipedia (2012) *The Way of St James*, accessed 9/2/2012 at http://en.wikipedia.org/wiki/Way_of_st_james.

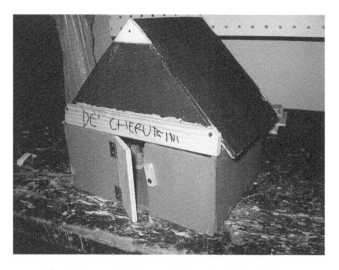

Sead's home. Photograph taken by J. Cunningham.

Section 1

Psychoanalytic Theory Interwoven with Occupational Therapy

This section weaves psychoanalytic theory back into occupational therapy. It begins with thinking about the therapeutic use of self and subsequently covers the major theoretical concepts in psychoanalysis by linking the work of Sigmund Freud, Melanie Klein, Wilfred Bion, Donald Winnicott and John Bowlby to current clinical practice examples. The final chapter in this section traces theory from the Fidlers' seminal work, *Occupational Therapy as a Communication Process* (1963), to psychoanalytic thinking in occupational therapy today (2012).

The authors have introduced psychoanalytic concepts to the reader through a brief description of the ideas and then applied them in clinical vignettes. Our hope is to make theory visible through the use of these practice stories. Occupational therapy readers are encouraged to research the original theory papers of Freud, Klein, Bion, Winnicott, Bowlby and Fidler, which may become a source of knowledge and delight as they discover within them a resonance to their own work and thinking. It is this use of theory that can illuminate and support the emotional work undertaken with clients.

Psychoanalytic Thinking in Occupational Therapy: Symbolic, Relational and Transformative, First Edition.
Lindsey Nicholls, Julie Cunningham Piergrossi, Carolina de Sena Gibertoni and Margaret A. Daniel.
© 2013 John Wiley & Sons, Ltd. Published 2013 by John Wiley & Sons, Ltd.

2 The 'Therapeutic Use of Self' in Occupational Therapy

Lindsey Nicholls

Much of this chapter has been taken from the introductory section I wrote for my PhD research (2002–2010). As my doctoral studies were within the disciplines of psychoanalytic sociology and political studies, the initial chapters were used to orientate the readers to the art and science of occupational therapy. As such, the 'therapeutic use of self' attempted to outline the concerns I had about occupational therapy's loss of 'wonder and delight' (Nicholls, 2007, p. 56) in the unconscious. I felt this loss particularly affected the therapist's ability to recognise the multilayered communication that was part of working with clients by paying attention to what was said, not said, done and felt (by the therapist and the client). This mixture of conscious and unconscious communication could offer containment (i.e. a deep level of understanding) for the patient and provide the emotionally honest support needed for clients to begin to consider making changes.

Finding a language and practice examples that would describe and explore occupational therapy for sociologists, psychoanalytic psychotherapists and political scientists was hard enough, but what I had not anticipated was the resistance I would experience when talking to occupational therapists about these concepts.

The professional imperative to be positive (part 1)

In my role as an academic staff member I had a 2-hour 'debrief' session scheduled with a group of undergraduate occupational therapy students. It was a Friday and they had just returned from 12 weeks of clinical placements to hand in their practice evaluation forms, attend the debrief session and hear about their future taught modules. The students were excited to see each other and there was a buzz in the workshop room as they shared stories of

Psychoanalytic Thinking in Occupational Therapy: Symbolic, Relational and Transformative, First Edition.
Lindsey Nicholls, Julie Cunningham Piergrossi, Carolina de Sena Gibertoni and Margaret A. Daniel.
© 2013 John Wiley & Sons, Ltd. Published 2013 by John Wiley & Sons, Ltd.

what they did on placement. I joined them, and after outlining that the debrief was a way of extending their shared learning, I asked them each to describe one situation they would like further thought and reflection on by the group.

Many of students raised the same concern: that of managing their relationship with the client. They said they wanted to be respectful, show concern (be client centred) and not overstep the 'boundaries'. What they didn't know was how to answer clients who asked personal questions, invited them to visit after they had ended their placement or told them a 'secret' (i.e. something they asked them not to share with other staff). They all agreed that these were difficult situations and many of the students felt they should be 'honest' and tell patients that they did not share 'personal information' with clients. When I asked what their reasons were for not disclosing 'personal information', they could only state, somewhat defensively, that they had been told not to. While this 'rule book' approach was being explored, a mature female student said she did tell her clients certain things about herself because she thought it would help them. She told clients that she had teenage children and believed this would help them feel they were 'normal' when they struggled with their children. She didn't want them to feel there was a difference between her and them.

When I suggested to the students that boundaries protect the patient from the therapist's less helpful intensions, the students seemed confused. They could not imagine that their goodwill and positively stated goal of enabling clients to achieve independence was not sufficient to establish a good therapeutic relationship. What they seemed to deny was that in any relationship there are many conflicted and unconscious layers of interaction and that they may have needed to consider the client's sense of shame and/or humiliation at needing help. These hidden or unconscious feelings could have been communicated by clients as an intrusive question or subtly seductive comments.

Had I known of the psychodrama work that Carolina Gibertoni had undertaken with occupational therapy students (described in Chapter 12), I might have asked the students to role play their interactions with clients, but I suspect that for this group it would not have been possible. They could not conceive of a less than perfect way of working with clients, and in their clinically reasoned narratives they positioned themselves as therapists who were conscious, well intentioned and full of hope for the client. What could not co-exist with these positive views of care work was the notion of an unconscious, something that is part of us all and affects our every interaction and choice of activity.

As Main (1957), in his seminal article 'The ailment', based on the observation of a long-term care facility, stated: 'there can be never be certain guarantee that the therapist facing great resistant distress will be immune from using interpretations in the way nurses use sedatives – to sooth themselves when desperate, and to escape from their own distressing ailment of ambivalence and hatred . . . The temptation to conceal from ourselves and our patients increasing hatred behind frantic goodness is the greater the more worried we become' (1957, p. 130).

Conscious and unconscious communication

In our considering a title for this book, it was suggested that if we used the words 'psychodynamic thinking in occupational therapy', it might be more palatable to the intended occupational therapy market, but it was a unanimous decision to keep 'psychoanalysis' as part of our focus in this book. Psychoanalysis, perhaps more than any other discipline, incorporates the notion of an unconscious into all that we say, do, believe, feel and think. Each of the authors has used psychoanalysis as a way of understanding patients, clinical situations, social environments and themselves. During my ethnographic research into the relational (i.e. emotional) work undertaken by occupational therapists in acute care clinical settings (Nicholls, 2010), it was deeply reassuring that therapists were acutely aware of clients' layered communication, which was difficult to access through standardised assessment techniques.

Clients' narratives had to 'felt', intuited and sometimes confronted so that a robust therapeutic relationship could be established between the occupational therapist and their patient. This relationship was based on the therapist being emotionally available for the client to locate their distress (or unconscious projections) in the therapist until they were ready to consider what these feelings could mean for their future life. This emotionally complex and rewarding work, while being tacitly understood in many clinical settings, had not been articulated in many profession-specific (occupational therapy) academic texts. The psychoanalytic occupational therapy model presented in this book (MOVI, Chapter 7) does consider the unconscious communication between client and therapist within the medium of 'doing'. The book has many examples of how clients' verbal and non-verbal communication is taken in by the occupational therapist and held (contained) until the patient can tolerate understanding it for themselves. The process of containment is central to the work that is done with clients using the relational model, the MOVI.

> Containment as a psychoanalytic concept involves the analyst keeping a space inside their mind that allows for the patient's projective identifications to be 'taken in' and processed. This act may allow the patient to feel understood, and if given sufficient thoughtfulness (a mixture of personal experience, theoretical knowledge and tolerance of these painful experiences) can be brought to bear on these projections, meaning may emerge.
> (Nicholls, 2000, p. 42)

Perhaps what is unique in an occupational therapy response, and different from an analyst who uses words, is that the occupational therapist communicates through doing and words.

This book, using the MOVI, explores how psychoanalysis, as a theory and practice, can allow occupational therapists to work with clients' thoughts, feelings and words through understanding their 'doing'. The emphasis of this chapter is on the occupational therapists' use of themselves in the therapeutic relationship. This 'use of self' pertains to a sensitive receptive capacity that therapists are able to develop towards clients. It often requires (as stated in Chapter 1) that the therapist has been able to explore difficult and painful areas in their past and present life. In other words, the therapist has had or continues to have therapy for their emotional well-being; it is this that allows them to do the demanding work with clients.

The professional imperative to be positive (part 2)

To return to my earlier example of the debrief with the OT students, when I suggested to the group that what may enhance their communication with clients would be a period of therapy for themselves, it seemed to be the final straw in my attempts to allow this group to think about themselves and the client. Students looked at me with a mixture of anger and dismay; it was as if I suggesting that there was something 'wrong' with them. They retreated into a sullen silence and the workshop limped to an unsatisfactory end.

It was only much later, in trying to think through what had gone so wrong in this teaching session, that I realised I had missed a vital step in the process: I hadn't first listened to them. I had expected the students to be able to hear and respond to the clients' unmet needs, identify with their disappointments and feel their pain. How could they perform that transformational role . . . if no one had offered that to them?

'The important thing is to connect'

Ormont (1988), in an article on the role of therapist in assisting clients in group therapy to recognise their need for (and unconscious defences against) intimacy, stated: 'In E. M. Forster's words, "The important thing is to connect." Nothing has caused more suffering over the millennia than people's inability to do just that. Psychoanalysis has from the beginning sought to help people overcome barriers towards themselves and others' (p. 30). Psychoanalysis uses the relationship established between the analyst and the patient as its primary method of therapy (Bateman and Holmes, 1995; Layton, 2008). It is within this relationship that the patient can gain an understanding of themselves and thereby begin the process of change. The therapeutic relationship can bring with it all the struggles, complexity and rewards of any close relationship. The responsibilities in this intimate relationship are both mutual and separate; the analyst maintains a constant thoughtfulness about the patient through a process of containment and interpretation (Ogden, 1979), while the patient investigates their inner world through free association and an exploration of transference phenomena. Although both are changed by the experience of (the relationship with) the other, it is the patient who is desirous of change, and the analyst who offers their capacity (self) for this intense engagement in a process of transformation or change for the patient (Craib, 2001).

Fidler and Fidler (1963) discuss how the relationship between occupational therapist and patient is *as valuable* as the activity undertaken in treatment. They refer to the transference and projections that patients may have with the therapist and encourage occupational therapists to consider what these relationships may represent for the client, and to consider this understanding in their interactions and use of activities in treatment. They employ the notion of an occupational therapist using the relationship established with the client as a legitimate therapeutic agent of change in treatment; they call this type of intervention 'the use of self in treatment' (Fidler and Fidler, 1963, p. 71).

Fidler and Fidler (1963) also expressed a concern that this emphasis on the relationship between therapist and patient may take precedence over the significance of an engagement in occupations as part of the treatment. Perhaps 40 years on we can see that this pendulum has now swung to an overemphasis on activity as the only real (valid) therapeutic agent of change, and the relationship between therapist and client has been underplayed in occupational therapy literature as a need for 'client-centred' approaches (Reberio, 2000; Sumsion, 2006; Townsend and Polatajko, 2007). The MOVI (Chapter 7) offers a rebalancing of the conscious and unconscious interplay between therapist, client and the doing of an activity. (Chapter 6 covers the development following this initial Fidler and Fidler (1963) work, incorporating the relational thinking behind the MOVI.)

Client-centred practice in occupational therapy

In the past decade a 'client-centred' approach to practice has been a basic premise in all occupational therapy applications. Its underlying assumption, which comes directly from the work of Carl Rogers (1902–1987), is that the patient (known as 'client') is best able to identify their problem areas and performance deficits and thereby indicate their therapy goals (Thorne, 1996). This type of approach is often framed in idealistic terms, but recent literature points to the difficulties in implementing these theoretical concepts in practice (Wilkins, Pollock, Rochon and Law, 2001; Reberio, 2000; Sumsion and Smyth, 2000).

The relationship established between client and occupational therapist is seen as having the essential qualities of a Rogerian approach to client-centred practice: the authentic response of the therapist, an unconditional acceptance of the client, and an empathetic response to what is brought into the situation of therapy. 'It was Rogers' contention – and he held firmly to it for over 40 years – that if the therapist proves able to offer a relationship where congruence, acceptance and empathy are all present, then therapeutic movement will almost invariably occur' (Thorne, 1996, p. 135).

This approach to working with patients was developed as a reaction to the more pessimistic and deterministic view of human nature that psychoanalysis was purported to suggest. The replacement of the term 'patient' by 'client' gave an emphasis to the self-responsibility the person (client) had in the relationship with the therapist. The value of the therapy was placed in the relationship that the patient established with the therapist, and this was linked not to the therapist's techniques, but to the quality of their interaction. This capacity of the therapist to be fully aware of and in tune with the client's world was the method of the therapy undertaken.

Before his death, Rogers accepted the shift of the term 'client-centred' to 'person-centred therapy' as a description of the nature of the interaction between therapist and client. He wrote about the feeling of 'presence' that he experienced when with a client. This, he maintained, was an experience of himself and the 'other' that was spiritual and existential in its quality, and allowed him a spontaneity of action and association that was often powerful and meaningful for the client (and himself) and led to fundamental changes in the relationship. Rogers maintained that he was able to offer people a 'space in which to find themselves' (Thorne, 1996, p. 123).

Rogers' approach was phenomenological in nature and practice, and although focused on the conscious experience of the client, his description of 'presence' echoes the discussion by therapists who work within an analytic framework and who are attentive to their 'countertransference' (Ogden, 1997, 1994) – that is, their internal response to the patient. I have wondered if Rogers' account of presence carried an echo of the experience of an analysis which leads to a deeper under-standing of the patient/client by using ever more sensitive listening skills, including listening to one's inner dialogue as well as the words spoken by the client.

In Rogers' explanation of presence he described it as getting in touch with something that is not fully conscious: 'the unknown in me, when perhaps I am in a slightly altered state of consciousness in the relationship, then whatever I do seems to be full of healing' (Rogers, in Thorne, 1996, p. 136). This altered state of consciousness may be similar to the analytic description of maintaining an attitude of 'evenly suspended attention' (Craib, 2001, p. 203) to the communication of the patient, where the analyst's unconscious is able to comprehend the unconscious communication from the client. The importance of the therapist paying attention to their countertransference will be discussed more fully in the subsequent section, 'Concerns with client-centred practice'. My unease with an absolute adherence to a client-centred approach is that it does not include the notion that a client's communication is not wholly conscious, or that we (as therapists) are less than perfect in our ability to tolerate the relationships with some of our patients. In other words, the client may be either unwilling or unable to tell us what concerns them, and for our own inner reasons, we may not be able to hear them or respond with sensitivity and/or an acknowledgement of their hurt or shame.

Telling myself first

A friend of mine, who had been through a period of considerable distress many years earlier, said to me one day, as if in passing, that the period of depression she had experienced had been precipitated by a rape. I was shocked and asked why she had never told me at the time. She looked taken aback and said, 'Don't you understand? I had to tell myself first.'

Concerns with client-centred practice

I think that a client-centred approach to occupational therapy has many merits, and when used in a context of disempowered communities and/or individuals it may well provide an equality in relationships which allows for enablement and trans-formation: for example, Watson and Swartz (2004) have written an account of this approach in South Africa. It was eloquently described in Townsend's account of her research into a clubhouse model introduced to a mental health facility (Townsend, 1997). My concerns with the overemphasis in occupational therapy on a client-centred approach as the only way of establishing a relationship with a patient is that it does not account for the way clients structure their stories to be understood by professionals, the layers of meaning and intent in what is said by the clients, the potential misuse of empathy in the relationship, and finally the importance of acknowledging the patient's unconscious communication as a way of understanding their life and experiences.

The illness narratives

In their book *Introduction to Psychotherapy*, Brown and Peddar (1991) describe different levels of psychotherapy, from the supportive and sympathetic listener (level one) to the resolution of conflicts through the use of the therapeutic relationship (level nine). Their description of the 'intermediate level' (1991, p. 92) describes the capacity of the therapist to see beyond the patient's words to their layered meanings. Balint (1896–1970), a psychoanalyst, ran a series of seminars for general practitioners (GPs) in the 1960s and said that the patient quickly learns what is expected from them and shapes what they bring to the consulting room: 'Patients learn the doctor's language' (Brown and Peddar, 1991, p. 97). Balint was suggesting that clients may tell us stories about their lives that they think we will understand.

The following example, which comes from my clinical experiences in South Africa, demonstrates the sensitivity needed to understand the patient in an area fraught with the potential for cultural misunderstanding and/or unspoken personal shame. The clinician was a sensitive occupational therapist, Elaine, who worked in the 1980s with 'burns' patients.

Sensing the shame

Elaine worked with patients admitted to hospital who had sus-tained severe burns. Many of these patients were black men and women who came from financially impoverished and politically disadvantaged backgrounds and had been living in informal settlements (i.e. squatter camps). These shanty towns were built from bits of wood and scraps of corrugated iron and were often heated with open fires or paraffin burners. The potential for accidental fires existed alongside the warfare that frequently broke out amongst rival gangs seeking to control the different sections of the squatter camps.

Elaine noticed that when she asked patients how a burn had occurred they often looked blankly at her and said they didn't know. She thought what was preventing them from telling her about the cause of the fire resulting in their devastating burns was the belief that she, a white middle-class person, would not understand what life was like for them. She said she learnt to ask her patients, in a conversational way, if their burns had been caused by 'a paraffin stove being knocked over . . . or an attack by "skollies"[1] . . . or . . .' and she would suggest the different ways that the fires could have been caused. By doing this she removed any sense of judgement and blame, and showed she understood the experiences of their lives. She said that when she did this, the patients, often with some relief, could then tell her how the fire had started, how they had been burnt and how traumatised they felt.

The stories of our patients' lives are layered with meaning, and this is especially true when the patient is experiencing a period of illness, disease or distress. Clients may come to us with a legitimate physical complaint, but its symbolic nature can create a window into their lives that, with careful attention, may help us discover the meaning of their illness. This was eloquently described in *The Illness Narratives* by Kleinman (1988). In a phenomenological study he explored the meaning behind patients' physical illnesses, many of which were devastating chronic conditions. In one chapter he described a man who had a chronic bowel complaint that was exacerbated during periods of stress. Although there is no space here to give a full description of the man's life story or the density of the understanding that Kleinman brought to bear on the situation, it seemed that the man, who would never fully recover from his illness, used it to communicate some of his loneliness and remoteness in relating to others. 'The pain was not a minor theme, however; it had the quality of a distraction, a part of experience that broke into his isolation by proving that he was real. And it brought him into contact with the only caring human beings in the city with whom he had developed a relationship: his nurses and doctors, and now a pain researcher' (Kleinman, 1988, p. 81).

Kleinman suggested that we look at symptoms within the context of the person's life. He described it as the interpretation of symbol and text, 'where the latter extends and clarifies the significance of the former; the former crystallizes the latent possibilities of the latter' (Kleinman, 1988, p. 42).

Communication between therapist and client is a richly textured encounter, and it may be beholden on the therapist to understand the symbolic and manifest content of the interaction. Therapists are encouraged to listen to the illness event within the client's life story, and not see the client as a 'hand injury' or 'right-sided stroke'. The

---

[1] 'Skollie' was a slang term used for local (often violent) gangsters.

patient's description of their life, interests and occupational performance problems will be lost on the therapist who sees them as a symptom without a context. The following example comes from some of my clinical work in London, in 1996.

The meaning of hearing voices

A patient of mine, who was living in the community and who had a long-term enduring mental health illness (she had been diagnosed with schizophrenia), once said to me that when she went to the community mental health team for her monthly appointment with the psychiatrist, he asked her if she was hearing her voices again. She said if she replied that she was, he often then prescribed an increase in her medication. She said, 'The thing is, no one asks me what the voices are saying.'

Her voices were very important to understand because, during significant periods of her illness, they were heard as her dead mother imploring her to kill herself and join her on the other side as her mother said she was very lonely. It was during these periods of hearing this particular voice that my patient became suicidal and battled to maintain her routines of caring for her children and maintaining her home.

A story without animals

In the novel *Life of Pi* (Martel, 2003) the author presents us with a fictional account of a young Indian boy (Pi) who, following the sinking of an ocean liner, is left adrift on a lifeboat with a Bengal tiger for 227 days. This story carries the reader through a series of adventures between the boy, the Bengal tiger, a zebra, an orang-utan ape and a hyena when suddenly, near the end of the novel, it gives us an entirely different account of what occurred on the ocean. This alternative narrative has no animals; the boy is adrift on the lifeboat with his mother, an ill sailor and a psychopathic cook. Both stories carry a similar plot: in the first account the zebra and orang-utan are quickly dispatched (eaten) by the hideous hyena, who is in turn eaten by the tiger. Boy and tiger then co-exist on the boat until they finally find land. In the second, shorter version of what occurred on the raft, the cook kills and eats his victims, until Pi kills him.

The reader is left wondering which account was the 'real' one and may have been challenged by a need to have a story that was comfortable to read and easier to understand (the one with animals) – certainly not one that includes murder, cannibalism and possible matricide. By doing a simple correlation between the animals identified in the first version of the story and the people described in the second, the orang-utan could have symbolised Pi's mother, the zebra becomes the disabled sailor and the hyena is the murderous cook, but what of the tiger? Was it representative of an alter ego in Pi, so full of rage and fear that he was finally able to defend himself and kill the psychopathic chef?

I was left wondering if the moral in the story was that the reader (or someone who listens to narratives) may only want to hear the things that are palatable to their minds. The question for me in the book became: on whose behalf was the story being told? In other words, if I could apply it to our work with clients, do patients alter their stories because they sense that as therapists we are unable to tolerate the reality of their experiences? Does some of this take place on an unconscious level, where both patient and therapist feel an unease, but may ignore the disjuncture in feeling by using platitudes of comfort and surety; and when the client withdraws from therapy, is it seen as 'their choice'?

In the book *Individuals in Context* (Fearing and Clark, 2000), occupational therapists are encouraged to lead the multidisciplinary team in the arena of client-centred practice, humming the tune (of client-centred practice) softly so that others 'will join in harmony' (2000, p. 7). These are strong and stirring words for occupational therapists who find they are a lone voice when speaking up as a patient advocate in a team discussion. But I would like to make a more personal observation of the difficulty in remaining client centred, which has to do with the therapist *not wanting* to experience the feelings of the patient.

The therapist, in being with the patient in a real and authentic manner, may come into contact with feelings that are disturbing and frightening. In order to protect themselves from those feelings, the therapist may unconsciously avoid any further contact with the patient, or make a remark that prevents the patient from saying anything further. Some patients are unable to verbalise their inner feelings and experiences, and by using a mechanism of projective identification place those feelings inside the therapist for containment and translation. Ogden (1979) explains 'projective identification', drawing our attention to the fact that the mechanism is first and foremost an attempt at communication. Like the baby whose cries need to be taken in (heard) and understood by the mother in order for her to respond to its pre-verbal need for food, comfort or warmth, we as therapists may need to take in and translate the messages from our patients.

Understanding this process does not only lie in the realm of psychoanalytic psychotherapy, and occupational therapists may do well to examine their countertransference responses to patients, as it is within the mechanism of projective identification that the patient can communicate their feelings and experiences that may not yet be fully conscious. Book (1988), in an excellent article on 'Empathy: Misconceptions and misuses in psychotherapy', states that 'empathy is particularly important in gaining access to the patient's inner world – a world the patient may be unaware of or, if aware, unable to conceptualize or verbalize' (p. 420). The response of being empathetic, he states, is being able to communicate to the patient an understanding of their inner experience. However, for some therapists this inner world carries a confusion and painfulness which the therapist attempts to avoid by using what can appear as an empathetic remark, but which the patient experiences as patronising or hurtful and therefore becomes silent.

Book (1988) uses a clinical example where a new registrar (doctor) encounters a paranoid patient on an in-patient ward. The patient is enraged at his incarceration and is shouting abuse at the registrar. The doctor, in an attempt to be empathic, says, 'I am glad to see you can get your anger out.' The patient hesitates, looks perplexed, and then angrily roars, 'You bastard! To be so happy that I am this upset!' (1988, p. 422).

As Book points out, the registrar had equated being empathetic with being unquestioningly accepting. This had blocked the registrar from hearing that underneath the patient's anger was his fear and helplessness. It was only later in supervision, when the registrar could look at his own feelings of fear and helplessness, that he could begin to understand the patient's unconscious communication.

It may be this equation of client-centred care with compliant acceptance of a patient's behaviour or requests that has created some of the difficulties that therapists find in the new culture of 'client-led' services. I believe it is this lack of understanding of the difference between 'client-centred' and 'client-led' therapy that has caused some of the misunderstanding in occupational therapy and prevented therapists from taking a more active intervention in patient care. Therapists must remain involved in thinking both 'with' the patient and 'about' the patient. It is the capacity to both feel the feelings of a patient and wonder about these feelings that can allow the therapist to make an appropriate response and a therapeutic intervention.

In teaching client-centred practice to occupational therapy students, I often ask them to analyse the following scenario that I took from an advice column in a woman's magazine in 1993 (a period when HIV and AIDS had become a new anxiety for many patients).

> ## Julia's problem or the problem with Julia
>
> *Julia: Last year I had a very brief love affair with a guy at varsity after a long-term relationship broke off. I did not expect anything to come of the affair, so I wasn't at all upset when he disappeared back home during the holidays and never so much as sent me a Christmas card.*
>
> *The problem is that now I have discovered he is bisexual. I am terrified that I may have caught a disease from him. I don't have any symptoms, but the mere thought of it is making me unhappy. I wonder if I should try to find out where he lives and write to him – but what would I say? Please help.*
>
> When students start to describe what they have 'heard' being said in this brief communication, it quickly becomes obvious that what Julia is requesting – advice on writing a letter to the supposedly bisexual man – is just the surface of a deeply layered message. Students begin to consider if 'Julia' is angry with the man with whom she had a brief affair; they look again at her statement that he '*never so much* as sent me a Christmas card' as a sign of her disappointment and frustration at his ignoring her. They then wonder if he may have been a replacement for her unresolved pain at the ending of the long-term relationship she mentioned.

> Beneath this hurt may be her unconscious fear that she is unlovable, and the feared infection could symbolically represent a deep flaw that she fears she carries into each new relationship. Through using association and reflection, the students are able to 'hear' much more than what is actually said by 'Julia'. This leads into their considering how they could or should respond to her 'request'; after all, she wasn't asking for an analysis!

The student class exercise described above has been a useful tool in looking at the limits of a client-centred practice where 'client-centred' implied staying on the superficial (or manifest) level of a client's 'request'. Responding to what someone has communicated in their between-the-lines or beneath-the-surface narrative can be deeply reassuring. Joseph (1983) said that as therapists we need to be able to distinguish between a patient's capacity to understand (i.e. seeking to know about something) and their desire to be understood (i.e. acknowledged for feeling a certain way) by their therapists. The same patient may desire these mechanisms at different times in the progress through therapy. My experience in analysis was that when I had been deeply understood by another feeling receptive mind, I could go on and try to understand myself.

On not liking a patient

In recent occupational therapy literature there are few references to therapists struggling with negative feelings towards clients. The discourse of client-centred practice makes it impossible to dislike a patient, let alone experience any kind of hatred or rage towards them. And yet we know, as partners, carers or parents, that it is quite natural to feel a wide range of feelings in response to another, and many of the less acceptable feelings we have towards caring for others involve disgust, hatred and envy (see Menzies Lyth, 1988). Finlay (1997), in her article on 'Good patients and bad patients', described how difficult it was for the occupational therapists she interviewed to say anything 'bad' about a patient or even state that there were patients they disliked. In our loss of a psychoanalytic discourse in occupational therapy, we have lost a language to describe, and thereby understand, our experiences of working with clients.

In a small qualitative study I undertook,[2] I was struck at the number of optimistic comments occupational therapists made about their work with clients and how positive they felt about their professional identity. It was as if there were no experiences of awkwardness with clients, no occurrence of professional unease and certainly no feeling of failure. It was this overwhelming affirmation that made me reflect on the loss of thinking about the 'other side' of experiences in the profession.

---

[2] Part of a postgraduate qualitative methods research course.

. . . what had been lost in the modern occupational therapy discourse is the incorporation of a shadow. With hope comes despair, with love hatred and with pragmatism a sense of bewilderment and confusion in day to day life. The researcher is not suggesting that occupational therapists now slump into the mire of depression and hopelessness, but perhaps acknowledge that in all situations, in the profession and in themselves there are unanswered questions, difficulties and periods of unease. By discussing the 'other side' of our experiences we may be able to engage in further critical thinking, and learn from each other.

(Nicholls, 2003)

Some professionals working in health care have expressed a concern that if we (as therapists) were to recognise the extent to which we feel with and about our patients, we would no longer be able to do the work. Fabricius (1991), in an article called 'Running on the spot or can nursing really change?', said it was the number and intensity of projections given to nursing staff by patients in an acute care ward that made the thinking about the work very difficult. Theodosius (2008), in her work on emotional labour in health care, uses the term 'therapeutic emotional labour' (p. 144) to describe the interpersonal and deeply reflexive work that nurses undertake to understand and respond to their clients' emotional behaviour or outpouring. This is particularly important when clients are seemingly irrational or abusive and/or make complaints, as presented in the clinical vignette of 'The complaint' (Theodosius, 2008, p. 142).

However, if we are to work as therapists with clients, to consider all that they do and say as well as investigating our response to them (i.e. our countertransference) as another form of their communication, then it is beholden on us as therapists to reflect on our experiences (or what Theodosius terms 'reflexive emotion management'; 2008, p. 201) to understand and help our clients. Daniel and Blair (2002a; 2002b) have promoted the use of a psychodynamic model of supervision in occupational therapy, emphasising the need for the clinical therapist to use their 'feelings to inform practice' (2002a, p. 237). The loss of explicit teaching (and evaluation) of the interpersonal skills necessary for this deeper level of communication in occupational therapy (or 'emotional labour' in the terminology used by Theodosius (2008) and Smith (1992)) is an area of development addressed in Chapter 12 and Chapter 13.

Although I have focused on feelings that are difficult to tolerate, such as hatred and envy, working with patients who suffer can bring us closer to an understanding of ourselves and improve the nature of relationships we have in all aspects of our lives. Supervision and reflection may also allow the therapist to remain in touch with the very desire that brought them into the profession in the first place. The hope that, by reaching out to the other, a measure of comfort, understanding and/or change is possible is surely the core of all the helping professions. I sometimes wonder if it is the capacity to endure the pain of living that can give some measure of reassurance to those who face the darkness alone.

Most patients with chronic illness, like the rest of us, live quietly and unremarkably in the daily struggle of living. Our pains, like our joys, are small, interior, simple. There is no great moment to the illness or the life. Yet illness, together with other forms of misery, sometimes brings a kind of passion and knowledge to the human condition, giving an edge to life. And for some patients with chronic illness pain and suffering have more to do with life – and specifically with that aspect of life which is dark and terrible and, therefore, denied – than with a disease process. Perhaps the healer and the family, like the historian of human misery, must allow themselves to hear – within the symptoms and behind the illness, especially for the complaints of those of us who are most ordinary – the wail.

(Kleinman, 1988, p. 86)

On becoming a therapist

Hoggett (2006) uses the word 'compassion' to describe the robust emotional commitment that public sector youth workers showed towards their 'subject(s)' (p. 154). Benjamin (1990) uses the word 'love' to describe a process which occurs between two people (e.g. mother and child) that goes beyond a (fantasy of) destruction or need for reparation: 'The outcome of this process is not simply reparation or restoration of the good object, but love, the sense of discovering the other' (1990, p. 192). I know my current university occupational therapy students are very suspicious of the word 'love', as they believe it is unprofessional to feel too much for and about the client. In the short story 'The Little Prince' (de Saint-Exupéry, 1974) the narrator speaks about love, but calls it another name; to 'tame'. This concept is discussed between the 'Little Prince' and the fox, who explains to the Little Prince that to tame meant to establish 'ties' (establishing a unique link with him) and that this was an art that had been 'often neglected' (1974, p. 66). He (the fox) says that if the Little Prince were to establish ties, they would have a need of each other.

This story provides a salutary lesson for all therapists to maintain the boundary of time as a function of 'holding' (Winnicott, 1956). The fox tells the Little Prince that he must come at the same time each day, so that the fox can anticipate (and look forward to) his arrival. He says to tame him (essentially a reciprocal process) they needed to recognise their differences (as fox and boy) and make a link through an appreciation of each other's needs. This seems to mirror Craib (1994), who stated that psychoanalysis allows for 'the formation of relationships based less on the illusion of common identity than on the reality of individual separation, difference and dependence' (p. 198).

This chapter may frustrate readers who were seeking a procedural approach to working with clients and I suspect this feeling is frequently shared by my students (as described in the early example). When teaching 'assessment techniques' to students, I suggest that they invite the client to sit with them in a quiet, private room and invite the client to tell them about themselves. I say that this will be sufficient for them to learn all they will need to know about the client, but more important than this gathering of facts and impressions is that it will start the relationship between the two because they are truly listening. This is not a simple process and many mistakes are made by new therapists who may wish to 'make the client feel better' or not worry as much, etc.

What these therapists may find harder to acknowledge is that these wishes are more to do with wanting to be liked by the patient than really engaging with what prevents the patients from getting better. This conflating of therapeutic goals with personal needs is explored by Casement (2006) and he has many examples of how his seemingly well-intentioned approach to 'helping' clients was patronising and prevented them from learning about themselves. What I have hoped, in this chapter, is to suggest that using oneself in therapy is an attitude of listening that allows the therapist to hear the real concerns and hurts that are often hidden in the client's talking and doing. As Foulkes and Antony (1984) so eloquently expressed: 'The language of the symptom, although already a form of communication, is autistic. It mumbles to itself secretly, hoping to be overheard . . .' (pp. 259–260).

Conclusions

One of our motivations for writing this book was to try and capture the complexity of working with the client in a therapeutic relationship through a process of: emotional understanding (offering containment), making interpretation (developing insight) and having sufficient space/time for working through conflicts. This holding relationship requires the therapist to become more aware of themselves and thereby the many layers of conscious and unconscious communication from the client (what was said, not said and done). Our concern was that in the recent renaissance of reclaiming the word 'occupation' in occupational therapy theory (e.g. Wilding and Whiteford, 2007; Whiteford, Townsend and Hocking, 2000) what may have been neglected was the process required to become a therapist and to offer 'therapy', which allows for a change to take place over time. We are hoping this book will address some of the aspects of this lifelong process of learning to be an occupational therapist.

References

Bateman, A., and Holmes, J. (1995) *Introduction to Psychoanalysis: Contemporary Theory and Practice*. Hove: Routledge.

Benjamin, J. (1990) Recognition and destruction. In S. A. Mitchell and L. Aron (eds), *Relational Psychoanalysis* (pp. 181–210) New York: Analytic Press, 1999.

Book, H. E. (1988) Empathy: Misconceptions and misuses in psychotherapy. *American Journal of Psychiatry*, 145 (4), 420–424.

Brown, D., and Peddar, J. (1991) *Introduction to Psychotherapy* (2nd edn). London: Routledge.

Casement, P. (2006) *Learning from Life*. Hove: Routledge.

Craib, I. (1994) *The Importance of Disappointment*. London: Routledge.

Craib, I. (2001) *Psychoanalysis: A Critical Introduction*. Cambridge: Polity Press.

Daniel, M. A., and Blair, S. E. E. (2002a) A psychodynamic approach to clinical supervision: 1. *British Journal of Therapy and Rehabilitation*, 9 (6), 237–240.

Daniel, M. A., and Blair, S. E. E. (2002b) A psychodynamic approach to clinical supervision: 2. *British Journal of Therapy and Rehabilitation*, 9 (7), 274–277.

De Saint-Exupéry, A. (1974) *The Little Prince* (translated from French by K. Woods). London: Pan.

Fabricius, J. (1991) Running on the spot or can nursing really change? *Psychoanalytic Psychotherapy*, 5 (2), 97–108.

Fearing, V., and Clark, J. (2000) *Individuals in Context*. Thorofare, NJ: Slack.

Fidler, G., and Fidler, J. (1963) *Occupational Therapy as a Communication Process in Psychiatry*. New York: Macmillan.

Finlay, L. (1997) Good patients and bad patients: How occupational therapists view their patients/clients. *British Journal of Occupational Therapy*, 60 (10), 440–446.

Foulkes, S., and Antony, E. (1984) *Group Psychotherapy: The Psychoanalytic Approach*. London: Maresfield Library/Karnac.

Hoggett, P. (2006) Pity, compassion, solidarity. In S. Clarke, P. Hoggett and S. Thompson (eds), *Emotion, Politics and Society* (pp. 145–161). Basingstoke: Palgrave Macmillan.

Joseph, B. (1983) On understanding and not understanding: Some technical issues. *International Journal of Psycho-Analysis*, 64, 291–298.

Kleinman, A. (1988) *The Illness Narratives*. New York: Basic Books.

Layton, L. (2008) Relational thinking: From culture to couch and couch to culture. In S. Clarke, H. Hahn and P. Hoggett (eds), *Object Relations and Social Relations* (pp. 1–24). London: Karnac.

Main, T. (1957) The ailment. *British Journal of Medical Psychology*, 30, 129–145.

Martel, Y. (2003) *Life of Pi*. Edinburgh: Canongate.

Menzies Lyth, I. (1988) *Containing Anxiety in Institutions*. London: Free Association Books.

Nicholls, L. (2000) Working with staff groups: Containment as a prelude to change. Unpublished master's thesis. Tavistock and Portman NHS Library, London.

Nicholls, L. (2010) 'Putting it into words': A psychoanalytically orientated ethnographic study of hospital based clinical occupational therapy departments in the UK and South Africa. Unpublished PhD thesis. University of West of England, Bristol.

Nicholls, L. E. (2003) Factors in mental health multidisciplinary teamwork that impact on the professional identity of occupational therapists. Unpublished research project. Department of Health Sciences and Social Care, Brunel University.

Nicholls, L. E. (2007) A psychoanalytic discourse in occupational therapy. In J. Creek and A. Lawson-Porter (eds), *Contemporary Issues in Occupational Therapy: Reasoning and Reflection* (pp. 55–85). Chichester: John Wiley & Sons.

Ogden, T. (1979) On projective identification. *International Journal of Psychoanalysis*, 60, 357–373.

Ogden, T. (1994) The analytic third: Working with intersubjective clinical facts. *International Journal of Psychoanalysis*, 75, 3–19.

Ogden, T. (1997) Reverie and metaphor: Some thoughts on how I work as a psychoanalyst. *International Journal of Psychoanalysis*, 78, 719–732.

Ormont, L. (1988) The leader's role in resolving resistances to intimacy in the group settings. *International Journal of Group Psychotherapy*, 38 (1), 29–45.

Reberio, K. (2000) Client perspectives on occupational therapy practice: Are we truly client centered? *Canadian Journal of Occupational Therapy*, 67 (1), 7–14.

Smith, P. (1992) *The Emotional Labour of Nursing*. London: Macmillan.

Sumsion, T. (2006) *Client Centred Practice in Occupational Therapy* (2nd edn). London: Churchill-Livingstone Elsevier.

Sumsion, T., and Smyth, G. (2000) Barriers to client-centeredness and their resolution. *Canadian Journal of Occupational Therapy*, 67 (1), 15–21.

Theodosius, C. (2008) *Emotional Labour in Health Care: The Unmanaged Heart of Nursing*. Abingdon: Routledge.

Thorne, B. (1996) Person centred therapy. In W. Dryden (ed.), *Handbook of Individual Therapy* (pp. 121–146). London: Sage.

Townsend, E. (1997) Occupation: Potential for personal and social transformation. *Journal of Occupational Science*, 4 (1), 18–26.

Townsend, E., and Polatajko, H. (2007) *Enabling Occupation II: Advancing an Occupational Therapy Vision for Health, Well-Being, and Justice through Occupation*. Ottawa: CAOT Publications ACE.

Watson, R., and Swartz, L. (2004) *Transformation through Occupation*. London: Whurr.

Whiteford, G., Townsend, E., and Hocking, C. (2000) Reflections on a renaissance of occupation. *Canadian Journal of Occupational Therapy*, 67 (1), 61–69.

Wilding, C., and Whiteford, G. (2007) Language, identity and representation: Occupation and occupational therapy in acute settings. *Australian Occupational Therapy Journal*, 54 (3), 180–187.

Wilkins, S., Pollock, N., Rochon, S., and Law, M. (2001) Implementing client-centered practice: Why is it so difficult to do? *Canadian Journal of Occupational Therapy*, 68 (2), 70–79.

Winnicott, D. (1956) Primary maternal preoccupation. In D. Winnicott, *Through Paediatrics to Psychoanalysis* (pp. 300–305). London: Karnac, 1985.

3 An Occupational Therapy Perspective on Freud, Klein and Bion

Carolina de Sena Gibertoni

Introduction

Clinical events have always provided, and continue to provide, life-giving sap. They are the tree of life. Human events are in fact so full of life, ever green, in our occupational therapy rooms that they are a primary source of knowledge, a text on which to reflect and work (Miller, 1989).

Yet the need for 'grey theory' emerges forcefully as if there were a need for a theoretical framework capable of incorporating into one precise thought the different meanings with which clinical events present us. Take the example of what patients make and construct in our occupational therapy sessions. What can the product, sometimes perfectly formed, sometimes crooked and fragile, and sometimes almost non-existent, represent? What emotional undercurrents are present, not only in what they have made, but in the whole sequence of events that gave birth to it? In our therapy rooms, sessions can unfold in the midst of frying oil, boiling water, stringing pearls, baking cakes, moulding clay or sawing wood. All this happens in the therapeutic space where two people, therapist and patient, share a stream of emotion flowing to and fro between four hands and two minds.

Many interesting aspects of our professional practice might not have emerged at all if we had not drawn new thoughts from psychoanalytical theory which created distance from a primarily biomedical role. Psychoanalysis has opened up new dimensions in understanding meaning within our complex clinical practice, and has helped to give strength and breadth to occupational therapy by creating new models with respect to its basic theory (see Chapter 7).

A key framework within psychoanalytic thinking is the relational model, which considers the human relationship as the main therapeutic factor. Attachment studies

Psychoanalytic Thinking in Occupational Therapy: Symbolic, Relational and Transformative, First Edition.
Lindsey Nicholls, Julie Cunningham Piergrossi, Carolina de Sena Gibertoni and Margaret A. Daniel.
© 2013 John Wiley & Sons, Ltd. Published 2013 by John Wiley & Sons, Ltd.

(see Chapter 5) and further developments from studies related to infant research and infant observation have all validated its fundamental role. If we take into account the discovery of mirror neurons (Rizzolati *et al.*, 1996) and studies on empathy (Hoffman, 2000; Gallese, 2003) and memory (Schacter and Tulving, 1994), psychoanalytical thinking has gained scientific legitimacy in the field of neuro-science (LeDoux, 1996; Solms and Turnbull, 2002; Mancia, 2006). In our practice, just as with other disciplines, there is always an attempt to integrate theory and practice. Continual discussion with clinical colleagues, and dialogue and debate with other disciplines, stops us from being short sighted and allows us to advance our (occupational therapy's) professional development.

In this chapter I will be focusing on three cornerstones of psychoanalytic theory – Freud, Klein and Bion – in order to explore how their thinking can be applied (i.e. used and further developed) in clinical situations inherent in occupational therapy. Their contribution to theory represents a new way and a big step forward in understanding the phenomenology that triggers the 'doing' element characteristic of occupational therapy. The concepts of free association, transference, the unconscious, object relations, projective identification, the container-contained model and reverie will be contemplated in the complex dynamics which develop between therapist, patient and activity, grasping all the richness that the flow of emotion gives. To do this I will be using excerpts from case histories, narratives gathered from my clinical practice, which will be linked to theoretical concepts from Freud, Klein and Bion. My use of these theoretical roots has arisen from a careful study of their original ideas. Therapists who are unfamiliar with these concepts are encouraged to engage with the recommended texts and/or attend one of the short courses offered by psychoanalytic training organisations on these psychoanalytic theorists.

Freud (1856–1939)

'Such was this doctor: still at eighty he wished to think of our life from whose unruliness so many plausible young futures with threats or flattery ask obedience'. Thus wrote W. H. Auden in September 1939, the year Sigmund Freud died. With his death ended a life dedicated to thought and the study of mankind. The legacy he left was the theory of psychoanalysis, a human science that is still relevant today and validated by the progress made in related disciplines, such as neuroscience (see Solms and Turnbull, 2002).

In 1935 Freud received belated but very prestigious recognition from the scientific community – fellowship of the Royal Society of London for Improving Natural Knowledge (known simply as the 'Royal Society'): the most coveted award to which a scientist could aspire. When he signed his name alongside Newton and Darwin's, he wrote: 'I hope that these honours will benefit the future of psychoanalysis and psychoanalysts' (Camassa, 2006). Not occupational therapists, of course, for Freud did not know of this new profession. And yet, here we are, ready to receive some of the valuable legacy from his brilliant early ideas, resulting from his encounter with Charcot: 'a brilliant man . . . no other man has ever exercised such a similar influence over me' (Freud, 1885). Freud's encounter with Charcot was followed by his stopover at the Salpetriere in Paris (from 1885 to 1886) and his visits with Breuer. Breuer related stories to him concerning his famous hysterical patient Anna O, considered by many to be the mother of psychoanalysis. It was with this patient, who was in treatment with Breuer, that psychoanalysis was born (Breuer and Freud, 1893, p. 21).

Anna O was an intelligent young woman of the Viennese upper class, whom Breuer treated by including narrative techniques during the hypnosis he used with her. As a result, Anna was allowed to narrate the content of her hallucinations and would come out of her induced trance, symptom free. The patient herself coined the expressions 'talking cure' and 'chimney-sweeping' (Breuer and Freud, 1893). These terms were an attempt to give a precise name to a cure centred around a narrative, through which it was possible to express and bring out all those memories that had brought on her symptoms – now termed the 'cathartic method'.

Freud decided to use the same method of treatment and investigation as Breuer and published, together with Breuer, *Studies in Hysteria*, which described how hysterics suffer from painful memories of a traumatic nature. The revolutionary aspect of these studies was the understanding that an exclusively mental state could affect physical processes in the body. The studies present a gallery of hysterical patients, each one a detailed case study showing the various stages through which Freud built up his theory: hypnosis, massage, and pressure of his own hand on the heads of patients, directing them on what they should talk about. This process was halted when his patient, Emmy von N., in a clear and aggressive manner, ordered her doctor to stop directing her: '. . . having told her to remember this the next day . . . she then said in a definitely grumbling tone that I was not to keep on asking her where this or that came from, but to let her tell me what she needed to say' (Breuer and Freud, 1893, p. 63).

It was Emmy von N. who led Freud towards the change in method that he was later to define as the 'fundamental rule of psychoanalysis' (Freud, 1911), namely that of the patient using free association and the analyst needing to have an attitude of free-floating attention (Freud, 1912). It was later, with his classic analysis of 'Dora' (Freud, 1905), that he was to consolidate the concept of transference, a concept which I discuss in more detail later in this chapter. Freud stated that it was dreams that could reveal the unconscious desires and wishes of his patients: as he had written in 1900, dreams were the royal road to the knowledge of the unconscious (Freud, 1900).

With a leap across the space of a century, I will now endeavour not only to find in the clinical practice of occupational therapy the 'fundamental rules' introduced by Freud, but also bring to life details from our current practice that link up with his subsequent theories.

Free association, free-floating attention

'Back then, the work arose out of the symptoms, and their solution advanced sequentially towards its goal. I have since abandoned that technique, finding it utterly unsuited . . . Now I allow the patient to determine the subject of our daily work himself, and take as my starting point whatever surface the unconscious happens to have brought to his attention' (Freud, 1905, p. 439).

Peter's steps

In the long, dark and shiny hospital corridor there is silence. From the doctors' and nurses' room comes the sound of chatter and the smell of food. I enter Peter's room. Peter, an 80-year-old man, is lying in bed perfectly still. His eyes are fixed on his right hand, which he turns this way and that. He sees me and opens out his arms, as if to say, 'Look what's happened to me!' Then he sticks out his tongue and mumbles something, holds it between his fingers as if to pull it out of its semi-inertia. Peter has had a stroke; he's lost his speech and the ability to swallow. He has been diagnosed with pancreatic cancer, but cannot undergo surgery because of his age.

It's his first occupational therapy session. I sit down next to him, introduce myself and talk to him. He writes on a notepad, 'You talk, I can't any more!' and he shows me the jars – yoghurt and baby food, one meat and another fruit puree. He can only eat smooth creamy things, he cannot swallow and he points to his shoulder where there's a wet patch on his pyjamas; he can't help it, he spills food on the right side. Then he skilfully draws for me a goose and nods his head up and down, as if to tell me that he eats like a goose: puts liquid food in, lifts his head up and back and sends the food down.

I tell him he is doing an excellent job of recounting his eating difficulties – his use of gestures, mimicry and drawing help me understand. I ask how he happens to draw so well.

He writes, 'I've always liked drawing, I do sketches for ceramic pieces.' Then he wants to speak, utters a roar, looks at me hopeless and helpless, covers his face with both hands and weeps. I take both his hands and hold them in mine. He wants to write. 'I felt a strong jolt in my fingers and then my mouth went stiff.' He looks at me, and I too look him in the eyes; he makes a sinister sound 'Maaaaam'. Again his hands cover his face, again that hopelessness in his eyes and his gesture. He writes, 'Last night I practised drinking', and shows me how he pours some water into a glass, slowly brings it up to his mouth and takes little sips, and the water does not drip down the sides of his lip. He wants to get out of bed to show me how he walks. I help him put on his slippers, he's a bit shaky on his legs, but he makes straight for the bathroom door. Then he returns and places his hands on my shoulders and looks me straight in the eye, as if to say, 'I can do it – did you see that?' I help him back to his bed. On the bedside table there is a history book. I ask if he manages to read; he roars and makes sinister sounds in a dramatic effort to utter sounds articulated in words: he slurs out confused sounds 'rrr-ead at nni-aaght'. Then he writes, 'the night is long and I think . . .' He quickly draws a narrow cobbled lane between two low walls covered in grass which winds its way up towards a hill. Then he adds the sea in the background and writes, 'St Martin's path'.

He takes a page from a newspaper with uncertain hands, puts a finger on a precise line, and asks me to read. It's an interview of a famous English singer, Sting. I read his words aloud. 'Newcastle has an extraordinary and occult power over me. My recurring dreams are invariably set there, in the old house by the river. Everything that I had deliberately shut out and forgotten resurfaces in the unconscious, re-opens wounds and it hurts. And sometimes it blossoms into creativity.' Peter covers his face with his hands as he listens carefully. Then he picks up his notepad again and writes: 'St Martin's path!' and with a pencil adds more grass to the walls, and steps, steps, steps. The notepad is too small; the page cannot contain any more steps. Peter stops with his pencil suspended in mid-air; he looks disoriented, like he's lost his bearings. I tell him that I'll bring him a bigger note pad and a variety of pencils, so he can continue the stone steps on St Martin's path. He seems to come back to reality.

I tell him it was a pleasure meeting him and that I'll be back on Monday at the same time. We'll have a lot of things to do together and we don't need words, we can do without. I'll bring a board and some clay for him to make whatever he fancies. He looks at me with bright eyes, alert, full of hope, and waves goodbye.

Almodovar's (2002) wonderful film *Talk to Her* is a good illustration of these concepts. In this film the two roles of the person speaking and the one listening are reversed, but the condition holds true, that of being together with the other, being two, where speaking and listening become the elements of being together. Both are indispensable in order for the therapeutic encounter to achieve meaning and depth. Listening to what is said and not said, in a dimension of free-floating attention (Freud, 1912), allows patients to freely associate. In our professional practice this transforms into things: the products of hands, of the encounter, of the interaction of two people, of two minds. From the very first meeting, our task is to develop and foster a climate of trust and safety which allows patients to let themselves go freely to their own flow of thoughts, reminiscences, fantasies, which can slowly emerge and, in our profession, take on a concrete form in what patients 'do'.

In the case described above, Peter tells his therapist about his dramatic experiences, using a pencil. Being able to follow his own thoughts without pressure or prompting, he communicates his mental states and free associations, and transforms them into a product – a drawing – that speaks without any need for words. The stone steps that he wanted to continue drawing, even when the page could not hold any more, perhaps indicated the unconscious wish to continue climbing up, the desire to live, in terror of death, perhaps as Calvino (1985) wrote, 'Steps like dunes pushed by the desert wind' (p. 98).

In a seminar held in Rome, Wilfred Bion, in reply to an analyst who asked what his position might be when faced with a disease like leukaemia and the expectation of imminent death, said: 'Is there any spark to blow on and rekindle into a flame, so that a person can live the life that is still left? How much mental capital does that person still have? Could that person be helped to use that capital or not?' (quoted by Tirelli, 2008, p. 3). The occupational therapist promises paper, pencils and clay so that Peter may yet fan his flame and live the life he still has.

Transference

Freud recognised the concept of transference to its full extent for the first time in the case history of Dora (see Freud, 1905), who after 3 months' treatment left him precisely because he, Dr Freud, had not understood the transference Dora had towards him: 'when she had her first dream, in which she warned herself to abandon the cure as she abandoned Herr K.'s house . . . the transference took me by surprise . . . and she avenged herself on me, as she wanted to avenge herself on Herr K., and left me' (Freud, 1905, p. 536).

Freud realised he had missed understanding an essential element in the therapeutic relationship, that of transference. He had previously believed that if the analyst could ignore this phenomenon, the patients would recover from these unrealistic expectations (or feelings) for their doctor (analyst). However, as he discovered with Dora, his disavowal of these communications led her to act out her unrequited feelings and leave him.

> What are transferences? . . . They are new editions, facsimiles of the impulses and fantasies that are to be awakened and rendered conscious as the analysis progresses, whose characteristic trait is substitution of the person of the doctor for a person previously known to the patient. There are transferences which differ from their model only in this substitution . . . others simply reprint unmodified new editions. Others are made with greater skill, they have undergone an attenuation of their content, a sublimation . . . Those are revised and corrected editions, no longer mere reprints.
> (Freud, 1905, p. 534)

The concept of transference would be developed further in the case studies that followed Dora's and was taken up and expanded in research studies by several authors, linked as it is to a multiplicity of meanings. *Übertragung*, the same term in German, has within it the following meanings: transference, communication, transmission, projection, displacement and transportation. Later it was Bion (1977) who highlighted the notion of transportation as 'the transit from one place to another, as if transference were an experience where the patient transits, that is moves, from one place to another' (Bion, 1977, p. 89).

By using an example from another case, I will briefly refer to Freud's concept of transference – an extraordinary discovery – in order to highlight how the concept of transference in our occupational therapy rooms can also be expressed through the use of materials. It is as if these materials become a means to 'transport' something; a means to communicate, transmit, project, remember, move and transform emotional experiences.

Michele's clay man

Michele is a young adult on the verge of a new psychotic breakdown. He does not go out of the house any more; he doesn't even leave his room. He smokes hashish and barely attends his weekly occupational therapy sessions. During one session he creates, with great concentration, a clay man; first the feet, then the legs, the body and the arms, and finally the head. His hands move fluidly, his fingertips seem to caress the various parts of the body that, little by little, take shape. But Michele's attention is focused on keeping his work rooted to the board: with each piece of clay his fingers move, shape, mould together, without ever lifting the clay in a vertical position. The end product is a small sculpture of a man, clothed, with even a cap on his head, who is lying down on his back on the wooden board.

'He can't get up,' says Michele in such a serious voice that it is impossible to argue; 'no one can get him up.' And he withdraws into absolute silence.

I suggest a few simple tricks, a toothpick, a piece of wire. But Michele remains silent. He runs a hand over his head, sighs as if in resignation and looks at the little man, motionless on the board.

'Nobody can,' he adds almost aggressively.

'Perhaps you're thinking about yourself, and about how difficult it is to get up!' I say to him.

'Eh . . . nobody can!' repeats Michele, and then, 'If I listen to you, he'll completely break, even his head.'

'Oh là là!' I exclaim with a small smile, 'but we won't be able to do anything good in this room! Is this how it's going to be?'

Michele looks at me, then he stares at the little clay man and touches its hat. He runs his hands through its hair, gets up and moves to the mirror as if to make sure that its head is still in place. The session ends here, with Michele leaving pensively and his clay figure lying on the board, put aside to dry.

What is happening in these sequences? What did Michele want to say about his small clay figure lying down? At the time he did not hold out much hope in our work together; whether I would have been able to lift him up, put him back on his feet. And his head, Michele's head? Could it have been damaged by me? It was a transference communication on my inability to help, shifted into a piece of clay.

This example illustrates Freud's thinking around the dynamics of the therapist–patient relationship that unfolded via this piece of clay; a concrete vehicle for communicating, transmitting, projecting and transporting. Freud paved the way for all those who have continued in the study and understanding of intrapsychic and interpersonal movements through transference. He also paved the way for occupational therapists to continue studying and researching the function of the different materials we use to help facilitate the understanding and communication of transferences in our sessions. With transference, the unconscious rules supreme and we can perceive it in many of the activities inherent to our profession.

The unconscious

Yet again, it was Freud's hysteric patients who trained his eyes and ears to grasp the logic of the unconscious, structured on desire and repression. These patients were usually young women whom Freud treated by establishing a connection between forgotten traumatic scenes and the symptoms caused by the repression of this knowledge. This was an unbidden resistance to recalling the childhood scenes that had triggered the need for a repression in the first place, leaving these memories to be forgotten. Freud showed that lurking behind repression was an inaccessible space, the unconscious, which contained the fundamental elements of psychic life – desire, passion, anxiety and conflict. Freud saw the unconscious as a realm of mental activity which can be accessed through dreams, wit and artistic productions. Psychoanalysis became the science of the unconscious. It is important to be able to access this realm in order to gain knowledge about the underlying causes for the symptoms that cause patients mental distress. Freud likened his method to that of an archaeologist, seeking 'to follow the example of those researchers who are so happy to bring the inestimable, though mutilated, remains of antiquity to light after their long burial' (Freud, 1905, p. 440). In other words, the work of a therapist is to make the unconscious conscious.

The patients who come to occupational therapy also have inaccessible spaces, the darkness of the unconscious, where there is anger, jealousy, desire, passion, anxiety and conflict; but it is essentially the materials used, together with hands, bodies, movements and the eventual products, that give us, as occupational therapists, access to a patient's unconscious mental life, as we continue along the vital path of the therapeutic relationship. Eighteen-year-old Elena, a likeable young girl with a diagnosis of borderline personality, is a good example of this process.

Elena's cellar

It is her last session before the summer holidays. Elena is working with enthusiasm. She rolls little sticks of clay, cuts them, moulds them again, makes them into strips, puts them one on top of the other. She rearranges them, then picks up another piece of clay and rolls it on the table with the palms of her hands, crushes it, turns it into a loaf-shape and sinks her thumb into the middle as if to form a hollow. She looks at her work as if from a distance. 'I want to give it a name,' she says almost to herself and then she writes on a strip of paper: 'Loneliness and Chaos'. She puts the strip of paper on the board she has used to mould the clay, next to her product. It is a strange composition, tangled, and extravagant. As if in a dream, Elena looks at it and starts talking of a sick rabbit, alone and abandoned, of dark cellars, of beautiful and strong women, of fathers who leave home and go to another house with another woman . . . Elena speaks as if she has opened the door to her cellar and has stirred up memories and thoughts from a dark space in her mind, has latched on to them and brought them back to the surface, there on the board, in the shape that her hands have given to her feeling of loneliness and her own chaos.

In the Milan seminars of 1975, Donald Meltzer said: 'If there is a series of events, and the child does one thing, then another, then still another, you need to make the same distinction that you do with a patient who presents a series of dreams and you need to understand if it is a series that is developing a certain theme, step by step, or if there is a single fantasy or different fantasies that are each abandoned because of the anxiety they procure' (Meltzer, 1975, p. 118).

Meltzer specified that it was important to pay attention to the way in which fantasies are represented. As an example he described a child who, during a session, played with Plasticine, making first one shape that he said was an island, then another that he called a volcano, then another that was a monster, and yet another that was a tomb. The way hands are used is part of the representation; hands are a means to make this representation – *they* create the stories (Meltzer, 1975).

Freud told us that there was such a thing as a cellar. He also told us how all his hysterical patients, who included Little Hans (1908), Schreber (1911) and Wolf Man (1914), each opened the doors to their own cellar. He also gave us an account of what these patients, rummaging through inner tangles, wanted to root out, bring to the surface and work through. Occupational therapists have the opportunity to help their patients open their psychological cellar doors through the sensory activities that various materials offer. Later in this chapter, I explain how Bion's (1962a) theory of beta elements changing into alpha elements demonstrates this move from formless sensory material to symbolic patterns of thought and words. It is the materials themselves that give us access; hands, bodies and movements create the narratives that flow through deep meanders of the mind and of the unconscious. The activity of *doing* can express these stories, communicate them and represent them.

How many memories expressed in the collage of our patients or in their personal picture books have been stirred up by the sight of a few images cut from magazines? Forgotten events, scenes and feelings suddenly surface again and come back to life on sheets of paper. How many memories are in a taste, which brings them out and anchors them to a dish of food prepared in a therapy session! Or even stroking and smelling a piece of wood, how many scenes come back to mind, thick with silenced emotions, thoughts forgotten as if buried in a drawer, but available to be picked out again and transferred into a shape that can express them!

These are the artefacts that we can read like stories, thanks to the 'fruitful contaminations' of occupational therapy's models in cross-fertilisation with Freud's theories. There is an opportunity for occupational therapists to draw on the key concepts and techniques that Freud theorised, such as the use of free association, transference in the therapeutic relationship, the unconscious, dreams as a symbolic language, the theory of sexuality, and the relationship between the id, ego and super-ego (1922). They have all become valuable tools for understanding and working through the dynamics at play in our therapy rooms. It was Freud who suggested that when we are working with our patients, our inner experiences (i.e. feelings and emotions) can put us in touch with their unconscious difficulties and painful realities. He was a brilliant doctor, who through his work as a neurophysiologist was able to intuit the difference between the brain seen as a physiological organ and the mind, the place where phenomena occur.

The dynamic vision of mental and emotional processes that followed this intuition has transformed the way in which we approach other people's pain: the relationship with disease has changed and the symptom has been substituted by the patient telling their story. The patient can speak and the doctor (therapist) is ready to listen, no longer looking at the sick body but addressing the person who is suffering and making requests. This extraordinary new way to be with a patient opened up a whole century of research, study and investigation on the construction of Freud's complete works. It is the fundamental assumption of Freud's legacy for occupational therapists: not a damaged limb to repair, not a function to be rehabilitated, not a body to be transformed into a technological machine, but individuals with their own emotional difficulties who ask us to help and light that spark of life left within them. And it is from this assumption that our professional rehabilitative practice draws its lifeblood.

Klein (1882–1960)

Melanie Klein's influential theories grew out of her careful observation of children. The basis of her work was formed by attentively watching the wordless acts and gestures of her children's emotional and sensory behaviour, picking up on signals which were the equivalent of language in adults. The scenes that made up their make-believe play were like dreams in the adult. Sandor Ferenczi (1873–1933), a Hungarian psychiatrist, was her first analyst and in 1919 he wrote a letter to Freud saying that 'a woman, Frau Klein, (not a medical doctor), . . . recently made some very good observations with children' (Grosskurth, 1985, p. 75).

Frau Klein herself wrote: 'During this analysis with Ferenczi, he drew my attention to my great gift for understanding children and my interest in them, and he very much encouraged my idea of devoting myself to analysis, particularly child-analysis. I had, of course, three children of my own at the time . . . I had not found . . . that education . . . could cover the whole understanding of the person-ality and therefore have the influence one might wish it to have. I had always the feeling that behind was something with which I could not come to grips' (Grosskurth, 1985, p. 74).

She started by observing her own children, Erich, Hans and Melitta, from a very early age. It was as if she understood their unconscious communication; as if they were speaking directly to her as she watched them. They seemed to be telling her about their experience with her breasts, about the inside of her body, their questions, their emotional movements and their needs. All of these she saw as vital to their growth. It was children, her own and those of friends and acquaintances, who made it possible for her to create her theories of object relations. She stated that, from the very start of life, babies projected and introjected in a to-and-fro movement laden with emotions connected to their experiences with an object, namely their mother's breast. This object (the breast) could be a 'good breast' that nourishes and rewards, but could also be a 'bad breast' that frustrates and disappoints. The latter experience created anxiety in children and, through unconscious phantasies of anguish, they pined, attacked and defended themselves. It was an experience of intense love and hate in the dense and intricate story of their relationship with this breast. This first maternal object was a central element around which children build their mental state and their relationship with the other-than-self (the mother and those relationships which follow). Klein suggested that this inner world, with its memories, desires and disappointments established by this early bonding experience, is used as a template throughout the person's life. In other words, it is used to give meaning to the events of the outside world (Klein, 1926).

Melanie Klein's theory was created through her analysis of children, observable through the use of a play technique. This was a form of 'free association' where the children could use any item in the therapy room, including the therapist's body, to express themselves. It was through play that she discovered, reflected, created and constructed her theory of the inner world of 'objects' that we all carry with us. The analysis of her own son Erich, whom she called Fritz, was the first case of child analysis that Melanie Klein presented to the Hungarian Psychoanalytic Society in 1919.[1]

In 1925, she was invited to London to hold six lectures on child analysis. She presented her work on child play and produced such a deep and extraordinary impression that Ernest Jones (1879–1958), an eminent psychoanalyst, later discussed her work with Freud in very enthusiastic terms (Kristeva, 2006). Following her warm reception in London, Frau Klein left Vienna and began her life in London, where her work (which she regarded as another child) and her fame spread rapidly. She remained in London, working and writing, until her death in 1960. Although there remains a distinct division between 'Freudian' and 'Kleinian' schools of thought, there are more points of commonality in their theories and understanding of human nature than is often given credit for by their followers.

In the following section I consider only some of Klein's theoretical thinking, and refer to those parts which have helped me to give meaning to the events of my professional practice as an occupational therapist.

---

[1] It is beyond the scope of this chapter to discuss Klein's ethics in using her children as case studies. As with Freud, many of her unconventional methods evolved over time into more structured endeavours. However, her theory on object relations remains a foundation for understanding a patient's phantasy life and their ability to form relationships.

Play

For Melanie Klein, like Winnicott (see Chapter 4), a child's play had a symbolic meaning, similar to the use of free association in adults. 'In their play children represent symbolically phantasies, wishes and experiences. Here they are employing the same language, the same archaic, phylogenetically acquired mode of expression as we are familiar with from dreams' (Klein, 1926, p. 134).

Play rules supreme in our occupational therapy rooms: children, adolescents and adults choose their activities. Motivation is an intrinsic part of choosing; it creates (with the therapist) an atmosphere of play in which anything can happen or develop. Unconscious phantasies take up residency in events that are condensed into a real object, a movement of the body, a gesture, a scream, a song, in a product that can take shape or remain unfinished. In an occupational therapy session, a piece of wood becomes a house; a ball of clay becomes a volcano; a button, the eye of a puppet; water and flour, a focaccia with rosemary. An open, playful atmosphere allows events to unfold according to what the therapist–patient duo set in motion, or what the therapist puts in motion with a small group.

Let us take, by way of example, the personifications that Melanie Klein discussed (see Chapter 7), which are very present in our sessions. In our rooms, as if in response to an inner need, children and adolescents, gather in small therapeutic groups, dress up and suddenly become witches, policemen, fairies, teachers, naughty children, cats, spaceships, cyclones, therapists and more. They improvise short plots in which the therapist assumes the role assigned by the patients, and play with the immediacy and spontaneity that our setting allows. Numerous emotional movements, projections, introjections and identifications intersect in their play acting, discarded and regained again in subsequent sessions. These sketches allow the therapist to understand what is happening in the inner world of the patient-actors and the whole group. This understanding occurs in the therapist's own inner world through the countertransference that is ever present in the speed and liveliness of the activity.

The internal object and the inner world

In 1957 Melanie Klein stated that only the introjection of an object that loves and protects the Self, and is loved and protected by the Self, can generate a feeling of integration that creates an inner feeling of safety, confidence and stability (Klein, 1957). This inner world is where the good or bad objects are placed: an object acting almost as a faithful version of the relationship the infant established with the breast. I believe it is in this inner world that we might place one of the functions of our professional practice, in an effort to modify or create a good and reliable substitute object, so that every emotion can be accepted and worked through. This subtle process of constructing a good object is evident in the therapy of psychotic children and adolescents, who show a quantity of excruciating anxiety unmitigated by any possibility to symbolise. Concrete objects and their transformations take on a particular significance because they are related to transformations of inner psychic processes. The possibility of attributing the characteristics of a good internal object to the figure of the therapist occurs through a process of identification filled with emotional movements. The following example is used to describe this process.

Fabio, aged 8, seemed to have internalised an object that did not transmit love or protection; rather it was one of constant rejection, unable to accept his projections. From the very outset of his therapy the main theme was that he felt he was a broken child, warped, non-functioning, something so second rate that you could only throw it away: he felt abandoned.

Fabio's broken Fiat

Fabio is sitting on the floor in front of a large mirror, his right hand holding his toy car tight, a finger of his other hand tapping the floor, in silence. Suddenly he begins to speak: 'The Fiat in the mirror is broken, the crane takes it and throws it away down the mountain. Let's throw it away Carolina . . . let's throw it away.' In a crescendo of anguish he gets up, runs to the door and goes out in a state of panic, screaming, 'It's broken . . . it's broken . . . let's throw it away.' He comes back into the room sobbing in despair: 'Carolina, throw it away . . . it's broken.' I try to reassure him: 'You feel ugly and broken and you are very scared that I might throw you away . . . but I'm not going to throw you away; in this room we can mend things that don't work very well. See, we'll try to mend the broken car.' I felt he needed concrete objects he could touch, see; words were not enough. At the carpenter's bench, just like in a real workshop, I set about pretending to repair the little car. Fabio's anguished sobbing suddenly stops, he moves over to the bench, climbs up and stands on a stool, carefully following the movements of my hands as I go through the motions of repairing. He seems to relax a little; he calms down and looks hopeful, as if he were asking himself if, in that room, there could truly be someone who accepted broken things, things that didn't work, and instead of throwing them away, eliminating them, would try to mend them. But it doesn't last for long. He gets down from the stool and, while violently hurling all his little cars on to the floor, kicking them, throwing them against the chair, shouts: 'Little children don't listen, they scream, little children spit, they fight, push, there's no place in the parking lot, there's no room . . .' I can feel his rage, the power and despair in his projections, and I try to act as a containing object that holds things together, reassures. I talk to him: 'You are scared that in this room and in my mind other children can occupy all the space and there's no room for children like you. But there is space. I am here waiting for you every Tuesday and every Wednesday. Here, let's build a parking space only for your little cars, so that they too, just like you, can always have a safe place.' And with some wood I begin to build a parking space. Fabio watches carefully, then climbs up on the stool; he doesn't dare pick up any tools but looks and follows each step. Then suddenly: 'Do you want the broken children? The ones who cry, the ones who are afraid of the dentist?' he says over and over, giving in to his despair.

I respond by saying, 'All children cry; everybody is afraid of the dentist. But we do grow up even if we are afraid; we become big even if we cry.' Meanwhile I take hold of one of his hands and guide it to help him glue a wall of the parking space and fix the wheels of one of his little cars so that they won't come off.

Our time is over; Fabio goes away drying his tears, thoughtful, with his usual runny nose. But he darts back in, picks up the toy cars and puts them into his box, closely side by side, almost as if it were he, Fabio, who desired such close contact, skin contact, to feel protected and held.

Slowly, over time and together with his therapist, Fabio has begun to hit nails with a hammer, glue plastic edges along his wooden track, try to paper the walls of his garage with pieces of coloured tissue. At first, these are just small transformations, opportunities to experiment, try his hand, test his abilities – modest and limited – helped by the emotional closeness of his therapist and by the motivation that Fabio transfers on to those objects: garages, tracks, tunnels and cars. Objects that represent in a tangible manner his need to be accepted, mended, reassured and held. Therapeutic moments created in the course of a long journey have enabled Fabio to tell, knead, cut out, glue, photograph; as if a good internal object were slowly peeping out in his desperate, violent and tormented inner world and had permitted him to have more faith in himself, the possibility of being, of existing, even if still 'a little bit broken'.

Projective identification

One of Klein's main contributions to psychoanalytic theory refers to the formulation of certain states of mind, which she termed the 'paranoid-schizoid (1935)' and 'depressive position' (1940). In addition to these structures she identified certain processes, particularly the concept of projective identification (1946), which is the focal point of much thought and writing in psychoanalysis today (see Ogden, 1979, 1992; Steiner, 2009). It is a concept that I have frequently encountered in my clinical practice as an occupational therapist and I think of it as an important part of the client's unconscious communication and thereby a significant factor in my work.

Klein became aware of the projective identification phenomenon while exploring the paranoid-schizoid position, namely a particular type of constellation of object relations, anxiety and defences (typical of the early life of an infant) which in some disturbed individuals can continue throughout their lives (Klein, 1946). Projective identification is a process whereby parts of the self, which are disavowed or denied, are placed into the object: that is, these hated aspects of the self are projected into an object, and then related to as if they belonged to that object.

The example I have used below is from Mauro, a young schizophrenic man who, in the last session before the summer holidays, attempts to expel the undesirable parts of himself, which are causing him pain and anguish, into me. It clearly shows how Klein's theory can give a new significance to the events in our occupational therapy practice.

Mauro and the rope that binds

Mauro arrives for his session on his scooter. His father, who precedes him in his car, has left him at the front gate. It's the last session before the Easter holidays. Mauro walks the scooter with the engine off into the courtyard of my studio, which is on the ground floor. I can see him outside fumbling; he ties a rope to the handlebar and then knocks on my window. He wants the rope to go through the window into our room. I take hold of the rope and wait for him to come inside. The rope has to be tied to my chair, to one of the legs, and I have to be touching it, holding it in my hands: 'Hold it, the thieves are coming.' The projection of feelings of persecution is so massive that I find myself looking out of the window for fear that there might really be some ill-intentioned person.

'I have to hold you tight this morning, Mauro. So many days without seeing each other, who knows what can happen! This rope is necessary to keep you close to me; it keeps us tied together!' 'Yes,' says Mauro, agitated. He remains standing. He moves non-stop back and forth from one end of the room to the other. He takes hold of his T-shirt, chest-level, and puts one hand on to his left ear. 'I must protect myself . . . I can hear the voices . . . they're threatening me.' Mauro often hears the voice of a woman, the mother of one of his school mates, a Ms Olga who treated him very badly when he was a little boy. 'You're thinking that I am a bit like that Ms Olga, treating you badly by sending you away for the next few days?' 'Yes.' 'But I'm here Mauro and I won't abandon you. I'll carry you with me in my mind and you're coming back here and we'll make pizza with mushrooms – what you wrote down in your notebook!'

Mauro sits down, once more grips his T-shirt chest-level, tightens his hand around it and pulls the T-shift away from his chest, telling me that he drives his scooter around his house but is scared of straying from the boundaries he has established: he can't go beyond Via Tortona on one side and Via Torino on the other. I say that I don't know his neighbourhood; I don't know these streets, so I can't understand where he has placed his boundaries. He stops and places one hand on his ear, the other gripping and pulling at the T-shirt. He sits down and picks up his own personal book lying on the table. He leafs through the pages and at the first blank page begins to draw some lines: Via Torino; another line, Via Napoli; then two lines that cross. Then he puts the pen down, hand on his ear and a lost look on his face.

I say to him: 'These lines are confusing; why don't we try with wood?' Mauro stands up, goes over to the workbench and takes a few pieces of plywood, cut-outs of different shapes. He grips one and declares it 'the church', then another, 'the garage', and another, 'the supermarket'. They remind me of his split-off parts, fragmented, like part-objects. 'Shall we try gluing them in the order you remember?' I ask him. He sits down and uses some glue to stick several of the pieces together on a strip of plywood, and then says: 'the garage, the church, the supermarket, the chemist's, here's the café where I go to have an aperitif with my father'. Mauro smiles. In fact, he laughs in front of his miniature neighbourhood. It's as if he could control and hold his neighbourhood in his hands, put together with the wood; as if he saw it and touched it all and could leave it there, in our room, to watch over and check up on me, who is going away, thereby eluding the feeling of separation.

It's as if his wooden object has taken the place of the rope, as if it holds together his psychotic parts and might placate the persecutory feelings he has projected so massively into me. Our time is over; Mauro unties the rope and throws it out of the window. His father is in the courtyard waiting for him. He goes out of the door, comes back in, looks at me and runs off; I can hear the engine of his scooter rumbling – to my ears, a cheerful roar in the courtyard.

The expression 'projective identification' is very broad and can present itself with different aspects. Some of our clients can split off from their feelings and project their anxiety or impulses on to the therapist in order to dominate and control the object. This unconscious operation can give the impression that the object is similar to the client and spares them any feelings of being separated. The object of the projective identification is experienced as an aspect of the ego itself that leaves its own body and comes to take residence in the body of the other. Using the mechanism of projective identification to deny separation (or difference) is explored in Chapter 9 on working with difference.

Idealization is used as a defence against persecutory anxiety and is its corollary . . . the psychoanalyst comes to represent in the transference situation a variety of figures corresponding to those which were introjected in early development. He is, therefore, at times introjected as a persecutor, at other times as an ideal figure, with all shades and degrees in between . . . Good objects – as distinct from idealized ones – can be securely established in the mind only if the strong split between persecutory and ideal figures has diminished, if aggressive and libidinal impulses have come closer together and hatred has become mitigated by love.

(Klein, 1950, pp. 46–7)

Thinking over the influence of the concept of projective identification in our rehabilitation work, I want to keep in mind Klein's considerations in her text, 'On identification' (1955), where this important phenomenon is seen as the basis for empathy. It is that very empathy, using real material in our therapy rooms, which allows us to share the feeling states of our patients, whatever their underlying illness or pathology may be.

Melanie Klein's theory and way of conceptualising inner objects accompanies me in the problems I have met in difficult therapies; with children, adolescents, young adults, parents. It has been especially useful in those cases where the pathology of the mind is so severe that it seems to refuse any possibility of a significant encounter or ongoing relatedness. Klein's thinking helps me trace back the clinical material, always referring it to the important events in the early stages of development, which affect mental structures and internal feeling states. The emphasis on transference, counter-transference and projective identification can help us look, and look once again, to see and understand where we may need to stop and change something in ourselves rather than in our patients. This questioning allows us to be as involved with our patients in the to-and-fro movements of projection and introjections, hate and love; in a relationship interwoven with the human and non-human objects of 'doing'.

Bion (1897–1979)

Wilfred Ruprecht Bion is the third giant of psychoanalysis on whom I wish to focus, in an effort to trace, in his thinking, those elements useful to our professional practice. He was both Indian and English, a scholar of psychoanalysis and a soldier, a doctor and a psychoanalyst, a mathematician and a philosopher, erudite and restless, often difficult and sometimes seemingly deliberately obscure. His thinking branched out in many directions; he studied not only the great psychoanalysts before him (and was in analysis with Klein), but had an interest in artists, poets, and myths. In mixing his two cultures, he contemplated the complexity of our existence; from the infinite and unknowable to the very essence of things. His writings appear to me, at times, as 'a beam of intense darkness' (the title of Grotstein's book, 2007) and at other times as 'a beam of intense brightness'.

> It would be nice, so seductive, if the mind, this archaic survival, could be so easily detected – but it can't. We don't seem to be able to smell it, touch it, feel it or see it, and yet we are aware of it . . . I think we could say that as far as mental life is concerned, we are in our infancy, we simply don't know what development is likely to take place or whether the development will be terminated by our magnificent equipment of simian capacity – being able to produce nuclear fission and blow ourselves off the earth before we can develop much further.
>
> (Bion, 2005, p. 6)

Bion stated that our mind, mysterious in its future development, is the scene of all our psychic impulses – from those primary and primitive, manifested in the sensory-affective experiences of infants, to the more evolved impulses, from symbol formation to representations in dreams and in waking life, and on to narration.

Thinking thoughts: learning from experience

For Bion, the mind is an apparatus for thinking thoughts. His model of the mind is conceived as a place where relationships emerge and move; described relationships of love (L), hate (H) and knowledge (K). These relationships can create profitable exchanges but also confused and disturbed ones – dependent, symbiotic and parasitic – producing 'thoughts that cannot be used for thinking' (Bion, 1962a, p. 84).

According to his theory, the first thought comes from experiencing an absence, for example the absence of a breast that is not there. Bion (1962a) stated: 'Is a "thought" the same as an absence of a thing? If there is not a "thing", is "no thing" a thought and is it by virtue of the fact that there is "no thing" that one recognizes that "it" must be thought? . . . No breast, therefore, no thought' (p. 35). Our psychic future (i.e. psychological well-being) is linked to this first thought, equivalent to an experience of a void, a 'nameless dread' (Bion, 1962b, p. 116). It is this formless experience of the baby which is communicated to the mother (caregiver), and through a process of maternal reverie, she (or he) is able to detoxify it, make it less dramatic and send it back to the baby's mind. It is in this process of communication (via projective identification with the mother) that, according to Bion, the first thought occurs: a primary preverbal thought, a primitive matrix of links between different sensorial impressions, one that is full of terror. It is the mother who makes this feeling of empty space bearable and returns it to the baby as a thought.

> As a realistic activity it [projective identification] shows itself as behaviour reasonably calculated to arouse in the mother feelings of which the infant wishes to be rid. If the infant feels it is dying it can arouse fears that it is dying in the mother. A well-balanced mother can accept these and respond therapeutically: that is to say in a manner that makes the infant feel it is receiving its frightened personality back again but in a form that it can tolerate – the fears are manageable by the infant personality.
>
> (Bion, 1967, p. 115)

Melanie Klein believes that a child's fear of dying is the first experience of a primitive terror of annihilation, and that a rudimentary ego – active from inception – serves as the agent of one's earliest defence mechanisms. For Bion (1962a) it is the mother who takes in the powerful emotions from the baby's primitive experience and returns them, detoxified and digested through what he calls the mother's capacity for 'reverie', to her baby.

> . . . reverie is that state of mind which is open to the reception of any 'objects' from the loved object and is therefore capable of reception of the infant's projective identifications whether they are felt by the infant to be good or bad. In short, reverie is a factor of the mother's alpha-function.
>
> (Bion, 1962a, p. 36)

For Bion, the mother is the person who *thinks* the child's experiences, transforms the content of the child's projections, and returns them having been thought through, thereby helping create the child's own ability to engage and transform their emotions and experiences. It is in this purely relational interaction that the ability to *think thoughts* is created: by creating a process that goes from disintegration to integration; this is the basis of learning from experience.

The container-contained model

In his book *Learning from Experience* (1962a), Bion describes the theory of the container-contained model, where the alpha function – the first relational task – refers back to the concept of reverie, as described earlier. The model of 'container-contained' has influenced many therapists who work with children and it struck me in much the same manner as those 'beams of intense brightness' I mentioned earlier. It is the thread that guides and accompanies my method of therapy with psychotic and autistic children, and adolescents with thought disorders, in mother–child sessions and in group therapy. If the container-contained model is thoroughly embraced in the continuous interaction between the two elements (the container and the contained), it can be transferred and applied to any context: like a framework that is with us in every therapy situation.

This 'beam of brightness' has allowed me to improve my understanding of what happens in our therapy rooms; from the patients' gestures, postures, movements, and choice and use of certain materials, to the therapists' inadequate responses or therapeutic impasses. I have thought of myself as a container, sometimes with leaks, holes or cracks in need of repair, a pot with a cover that does not do its job very well.

In our particular form of therapy, sensory elements are often manifested in a raw, bulky form without thought – what Bion would have termed 'beta elements'. These are the formless sensory experiences (mentioned earlier as a 'nameless dread') that can be so frightening for the infant or child. The therapists take on the function of reverie and help transform these beta elements into something that has meaning that can be stored and recalled: in other words, transformed into alpha elements. These can be in the form of thoughts, symbolic actions and/or words. Containment takes on the function of holding together shapeless parts or fragments, primitive modalities and proto thoughts; initiating a process that gives form to the formless. It is a good container in constant interaction with its content.

Rosalia's biscuit baking

Rosalia, a psychotic child, while making biscuits during cookery activities, throws flour up in the air, spills water on the floor instead of pouring it into the circle-shape on the table, upsets the bag of sugar on to the chair, takes a few bites out of the butter, and stands up on the stool. It's as if she were externalising split and confused modalities, beta elements, which can only be evacuated. I respond by saying, 'Wow! How frightened Rosalia is: scared of this room, scared of the flour, of the egg, the butter, the oven, scared of putting all these things together, scared of not knowing how to make biscuits!'

Rosalia gets down from the stool and starts running around, squealing and jumping about. I pick up the sugar, the flour and the butter, and once again prepare the flour well on the table – a sort of volcano made of flour with a crater in its centre – and, looking at her, I start singing: 'I've lost a little sheep tra-la-la . . . I've lost a little sheep . . . tra-la-la! She has a pink skirt . . . tra-la-la.' Rosalia stops and pulls at her skirt . . . 'And little blue shoes . . . and a green top . . . tra-la-la.' Rosalia goes over to the mirror, looks at herself carefully, and turns round to look at me quizzically. I continue singing: 'She has black curly hair . . . tra-la-la.' Rosalia laughs, takes hold of a lock of her hair and tugs at it, and lies down on a large pillow as if waiting for another verse.

Meanwhile I put together water and flour, butter and sugar, and sing: 'Such a shame to have lost her . . . tra-la-la . . . she wanted to break the egg, tra-la-la, and make biscuits, tra-la-la, . . . and put them in the oven, tra-la-la . . .' Rosalia gets up from the pillow and moves over to the table while I break an egg; she looks at me and laughs as if sharing a joke. 'But perhaps I have found her again . . . tra-la-la . . . Oh yes, I have found her again, her name is Rosalia, tra-la-la-la-la! . . . How lucky, I have found my little sheep. I wonder where she went!!!'

I start to knead the pastry and give a piece to Rosalia, who touches it and sticks her fingers in it, pinches a piece off and puts it in her mouth, another pinch and another bite, until she finishes it. 'My, how hungry this little sheep is! So hungry, that she can't even wait for the pastry to become a biscuit!' Rosalia looks at me amused and takes pinches from the pastry I'm flattening out on the table with a rolling pin. Next to the pastry, there is a shorter rolling pin for children. I cut off a piece from my rolled pastry and put it on the table in front of Rosalia: 'Carolina rolls out her pastry with the giant rolling pin, Rosalia rolls out hers with the little rolling pin.' Rosalia picks it up but swings it above her head. I help Rosalia by putting the rolling pin on the pastry and, with my hands on hers, together we roll it out to make it thinner. It looks like a little pizza.

Rosalia is constantly on the verge of stealing a little piece, but refrains; she doesn't do it. She looks at me and we go and turn on the oven. She skips around the table, goes to the oven, opens it and closes it, goes back to the table and pokes the pastry with a finger, so now it looks like a flat cake with holes. 'Yum, what a nice biscuit!' I say. 'Now we can put it in the oven.' And we do this. Rosalia stands in front of the oven and looks through the glass pane of the oven door. I pick up a book and sit next to Rosalia and the oven. And while the biscuit is cooking, I read.

It's the story of a little girl, Zeralda, who seduces a bad giant with her good cooking and makes him become a good giant and even marries him. Rosalia comes closer, sits next to me and follows the story without missing a single word or illustration. A wonderful smell of biscuits fills the room. The time is over; the biscuit is baked, golden and fragrant. But it's too hot, and Rosalia would like to wait for it to cool while we read the story of Zeralda again. But the session time is over; we wrap the biscuit in foil paper, and Rosalia takes it and goes away with it. She skips, goes through the door, pushes aside a little boy who is about to come in, comes back, looks at me, and looks at the little boy. 'I'll see you Friday, Rosalia, and we'll read the story of Zeralda,' I say to her. I can hear her mother asking what is in the foil paper. But Rosalia does not answer. I hear their steps in the courtyard.

No memory, no desire

Perhaps the most often-quoted part of Bion's theory is that the therapist should approach their work with a patient 'without memory or desire' (1970, 1992). This seems a strange attitude for a therapist to have when many of us, as government-employed health care workers, are asked to provide evidence of our work with clients by producing agreed goals within a time-limited treatment plan. Bion's concern was that if a therapist was sure of where the patient needed to go, they would not listen to what was important: 'it is easier to "forget" what you know and "forget" what you want, get rid of your desires, anticipations and also your memories so that there will be a chance of hearing these very faint sounds that are buried in this mass of noise' (Bion, 2005, p. 17).

Bion believed that it was with a quiet mind that the therapist could observe and make contact with the unconscious communication of the patient. This process allowed for the therapist to take in the communication and allow for new thoughts to form (i.e. the container-contained function of therapy): 'give yourself a chance to observe the growth of a germ of an idea. That is the fascination of this job; if one can get through to a fact, it takes a lot of believing – no fiction can touch it' (Bion, 2005, p. 18). Bion was suggesting that knowledge gained in this manner was a deep truth, gained through a process of dialogue and reflection.

Bion's daughter, Parthenope, linked this concept to her father's childhood in India, where culture and customs – the influence of religion and Hindu myths – transmitted an attitude towards life of hopeful, patient waiting. Parthenope Bion (1996) showed how this patient attitude was embedded in the culture and lifestyle when she used the example of a means of transport with which Bion as a child was familiar: the elephant. These animals are, after all, slow, patient, surefooted beasts: 'there were two elephants that belonged to our family, and I even know their names – that's how important they were. We would load everything onto the elephants, even the small folding harmonium that my grandmother used to play hymns every evening' (Bion, 1996).

Bion's concept of waiting without memory and without desire means that within the concentration that a session requires, the therapist does not need to remember what a patient said the day before, or what happened, and does not have to think over the meaning of the dream told by the patient, or wish a speedy recovery for the patient. These are irrelevant and disturbing noises that keep the mind from focusing on what is happening at that moment.

Pasqualino's pinchy-pinchy music

Pasqualino floods the room with noise. His only way to be in the therapy room is to look for sources of noise that can best defend him from me. Small musical instruments are ignored: he uses his fingernails to scratch different surfaces; small objects – like wooden ladles – he beats against the doors, walls and table. With pricked ears and tilted head, he listens to the sounds he produces. He never looks at me; 10 minutes into the session, he goes out of the room, picks up his coat and leaves. At first I would simply tell him that I understood how scared he was in that new space, with a person he did not know, and how he preferred to be on his own with his noises. I would ask him to give me his noises, his fear; I would hold out my two hands as if he could really hand them over to me. Pasqualino would stop a moment, sneak a look at me, turn round and immediately start wandering about the room, focusing only on looking for surfaces that might provide different noises to keep him safe. At times he seemed to be examining the space that was surrounding him in order to flood it and wrap it up with his noises, as if to control it and imprison it.

I had introduced some sounds. There was a metal triangle, which I would now and then hit with its striker, letting the sound slowly fade before doing it again; at times I would tape it along with Pasqualino's noises. He would stop and seemed to listen, but not for long, only a few seconds. He always immediately returned to his wandering around the room – distant, banging his ladle everywhere. I experimented with new elements, playing with water, little cakes, popcorn, soap bubbles. All with the same results: Pasqualino would come closer, seem to look, move away, start his banging all around the room and then disappear, as if to say I hadn't understood one little bit about him.

And it was true. I was activating memory and desire, resulting in Pasqualino's leaving.

He could not accept new experiences which were not extensions of his own experiences: I did not react as his mirror image. I had to transform myself into the sensory quality that he was using; maybe I would be able to reach him if I placed myself at his level, at the level of his need to feel wrapped by the same sensory material he was producing – noise.

A string of little coloured lights help me to define rather unconventionally the boundaries of a house-space inside the therapy room. I begin to stay in this little house, sitting on the floor, with a kitchen ladle, a triangle, a tape recorder. Pasqualino bangs his ladle against the wall and I reply by banging my ladle against the wall too. And while I'm banging I sing. I sing of how frightened he is, how he feels lonely and not understood, how difficult it is to be in that room, alone and with a Carolina who does not understand anything about him.

Pasqualino moves closer and then runs away; it seems to me that his attention span is increasing; he stops and opens his eyes wide when he listens to the tape of me singing, accompanied by our banging ladles. But what he seems to like best is a nursery rhyme: 'pinchy-pinchy triangle . . . the death of Striangle . . .' I keep time while I sing by lightly pinching the tips of my fingers, not daring to touch his. Pasqualino moves strangely about the room, spins, wiggles his fingers; he comes closer, then runs away, returns and runs away again. I understand that this game intrigues him. It is a tactile-auditory game with musical characteristics, more evolved than his game but with his own initial modalities.

Repeating this song-rhyme, keeping time and rhythm with my fingers, was like creating a way to be together; something that Pasqualino was able to internalise.

'When you have forgotten all that you can about your patient – who will do his best to remind you – then you may have a chance of penetrating this impressive caesura of knowledge, facts, and a chance of hearing these very small things that are so difficult to hear or see' (Bion, 2005, p. 18).

All of Bion's thoughts, the key themes of his works – from the technique with his patients to groups, from alpha function to container-contained, from the grid to the reformulation of Kleinian thought in the famous triad of L (love), H (hate) and K (knowledge) – are difficult concepts and at times confusing. It seems impossible that they might be useful in our profession. But, as I have already expressed, some of his thinking, which I have read and read again in order to try and grasp its essence, has enlightened me. I am referring in particular to the alpha function and beta elements, the container-contained configuration and his thinking on group work, which I hope to write about in the future. The emotional movements that we learn to decipher better via the application of his theories may assist occupational therapists to open their minds to new thoughts. Bion (1980) wrote: 'I have suggested this: discard your memory, discard the future tense of your desire; forget them both, both what you knew and what you want, to leave a space for a new idea. A thought, an idea unclaimed, may be floating around the room searching for a home' (p. 11). In other words, there may be new thoughts in search of a thinker!

Conclusions

In this chapter I have tried to describe, through the use of clinical situations, the influence of the psychoanalytical thinking of Freud, Klein and Bion on the comprehension of what happens in the occupational therapy process. Their precious contribution transforms our theory and our practice into an articulated, complex and interesting therapeutic form, capable of promoting change and generating new thoughts both in patients and in ourselves as occupational therapists.

References

Almodovar, P. (2002) *Talk to Her* (dir. by P. Almodovar; Spanish title *Hable con Ella*), distributed by Sony Picture Classics.

Auden, W. H. (1939) In memory of Sigmund Freud. In *Another Time*. London: Random House.

Bion Talamo, P. (1996) L'apporto di Bion alla psicoanalisi. Seminar 11 December. La Sapienza University, Rome.

Bion, W. R. (1962a) *Learning from Experience*. London: Heinemann.

Bion, W. R. (1962b) A theory of thinking. In W. R. Bion, *Second Thoughts: Selected Papers of Psycho analysis*. London: Heinemann, 1967.

Bion, W. R. (1967) *Second Thoughts: Selected Papers of Psychoanalysis*. London: Heinemann.

Bion, W. R. (1970) *Attention and Interpretation*. London: Tavistock.

Bion, W. R. (1977) *A Memoir of the Future: Book 3 The Dawn of Oblivion*. Rio de Janeiro: Imago Editora Ristampa.

Bion, W. R. (1980) *Bion in New York and São Paulo*. Perthshire: Clunie Press.

Bion, W. R. (1992) *Cogitations* (ed. Francesca Bion). London: Karnac.

Bion, W. R. (2005) *The Tavistock Seminars [1976–1979]* London: Karnac. Appendix B, 'Interview by Anthony G. Banet, Jr' first appeared in *Group and Organization Studies*, 1 (3), 268–285.

Breuer, J., and Freud, S. (1893) On the psychical mechanism of hysterical phenomena. In *The Standard Edition of the Complete Psychological Works of Sigmund Freud* (Vol. II, 1893–1895): *Studies on Hysteria*. London: Hogarth Press and the Institute of Psychoanalysis, 1955.

Calvino, I. (1985) *Lezioni Americane*. Milan: Garzanti, 1988.

Camassa, P. (2006) Il dottor Freud. Società Psicoanalitica Italiana, SPIWEB.it.

Freud, S. (1885) Letter to Martha Bernays (1885). In *Letters of Sigmund Freud*. London: Hogarth Press, 1970.

Freud, S. (1900) *Interpretation of Dreams*. Oxford: Oxford University Press, 1999.

Freud, S. (1905) Fragment of an analysis of hysteria (Dora). In *The Penguin Freud Reader* (pp. 435–540). Harmondsworth: Penguin, 2006.

Freud, S. (1909) Analysis of a phobia in a five-year-old boy. In *The Standard Edition of the Complete Psychological Works of Sigmund Freud* (Vol. X, pp. 1–150): *Two Case Histories ('Little Hans' and the 'Rat Man')*. London: Hogarth Press and Institute of Psychoanalysis, 1955.

Freud, S. (1911) The handling of dream-interpretation in psycho-analysis. In *The Standard Edition of the Complete Psychological Works of Sigmund Freud* (Vol. XII, pp. 89–96): *The Case of Schreber, Papers on Technique and Other Works*. London: Hogarth Press, 2000.

Freud, S. (1912) Recommendations to physicians practising psycho-analysis. In *The Standard Edition of the Complete Psychological Works of Sigmund Freud* (Vol. XII, pp. 109–120). London: Hogarth Press, 1953.

Freud, S. (1914) *The Wolfman and Other Cases*. Harmondsworth: Penguin, 2003.

Freud, S. (1922) Preface to Raymond De Saussure's *The Psycho-Analytic Method*. In *The Standard Edition of the Complete Psychological Works of Sigmund Freud* (Vol. XIX, pp. 281–284): *The Ego and the Id*. London: Hogarth Press, 1962.

Gallese, V. (2003) The roots of empathy: The shared manifold hypothesis and the neural basis of intersubjectivity. *Psychopathology*, 36 (4), 171–180.

Grosskurth, P. (1985) *Melanie Klein: Her World and her Work*. London: Hodder & Stoughton.

Grotstein, J. S. (2007) *'A Beam of Intense Darkness': Wilfred Bion's Legacy to Psychoanalysis*. London: Karnac.

Hoffman, M. L. (2000) *Empathy and Moral Development*. Cambridge: Cambridge University Press.

Klein, M. (1926) The psychological principles of infant analysis. *International Journal of Psycho-Analysis*, 8, 25–37.

Klein, M. (1935) A contribution of the psychogenesis of manic-depressive states. *International Journal of Psycho-Analysis*, 16, 145–174.

Klein, M. (1940) Mourning and its relation to manic-depressive states. *International Journal of Psychoanalysis*, 21, 125–153.

Klein, M. (1946) Notes on some schizoid mechanisms. *International Journal of Psychoanalysis*, 27, 99–110.

Klein, M. (1950) On the criteria for the termination of a psycho-analysis. *International Journal of Psychoanalysis*, 31, 78–80.

Klein, M. (1955) On identification. In M. Klein, P. Heimann and R. Money-Kyrle (eds), *New Directions in Psycho-Analysis* (pp. 309–345). London: Tavistock.

Klein, M. (1957) *Envy and Gratitude and Other Works 1946–1963* (pp. 176–235). London: Virago.

Kristeva, J. (2006) *Melanie Klein: La madre, la follia*. Rome: Donzelli Editori.

LeDoux, J. (1996) *The Emotional Brain: The Mysterious Underpinnings of Emotional Life*. New York: Simon & Schuster.

Mancia, M. (2006) *Psychoanalysis and Neuroscience*. Milan: Springer.

Meltzer, D. (1975) *Seminari Milanesi. Quaderni di Psicoterapia Infantile*, 2, Borla, Perugia, 1982.

Miller, L. (1989) Introduction. In L. Miller, M. Rustin and J. Shuttleworth (eds), *Closely Observed Infant* (pp. 1–4). London: Duckworth.

Ogden, T. H. (1979) On projective identification. *International Journal of Psycho-Analysis*, 60, 357–373.

Ogden, T. H. (1992) *Projective Identification and Psychotherapeutic Technique*. London: Karnac.

Rizzolati, G., *et al.* (1996) Premotor cortex and recognition of motor actions. *Cognitive Brain Research*, 3 (2), 131–141.

Schacter, D. L., and Tulving, E. (1994) What are the memory systems of 1994? In D. L. Schacter and E. Tulving (eds), *Memory Systems 1994* (pp. 1–38). Cambridge, MA: MIT Press.

Solms, M., and Turnbull, O. (2002) *The Brain and the Inner World: An Introduction to the Neuroscience of Subjective Experience*. New York: Other Press.

Steiner, R. (2009) On understanding projective identification in the treatment of psychotic states of mind. *International Journal of Psychoanalysis*, 90, 1435–1437.

Tirelli, L. Carbone (2008) *Bion e la psicoanalisi infantile*. Rome: Il Pensiero Scientifico Editore.

4 The Function of 'Doing' in the Intermediate Space: Donald Winnicott and Occupational Therapy

Julie Cunningham Piergrossi

Introduction

I am fascinated by the thoughts of psychoanalysts who theorise about spaces and space. They write about our inner space, full of thoughts, memories, emotions and imagination, but also about the space between ourselves and others, and our use of this space in a way that permits growth and useful learning for living. In this shared space we learn about ourselves and we also learn about others and the relationships between the two, about what it means to 'stick together' – as Pooh puts it to Christopher Robin in the poem by A. A. Milne (1927).

I remember being struck by the British psychoanalyst Donald W. Winnicott's (1971) description of intermediate space in human development and how it seemed so clear to me. The idea of a protective space that permitted closeness had a special significance for me, and I began to understand it more fully as I wrote this chapter. I realised that an essential part of (and struggle for) me was wanting to be close to others but at the same time desiring my own space and wanting others to have their own spaces and to respect mine. Inhabiting the intermediate space, as described by Winnicott, made me feel at home and comfortable, neither too close to nor too far from the others in my life. I believe that being aware of this in my 'self' and in my relationships has been very helpful in my work as an occupational therapist with disturbed children and their families.

Ogden (2001), whom I only discovered recently, helped me to understand how I had been able to use Winnicott's writing in the therapeutic story I will present in this chapter. Ogden describes Winnicott's way of writing as a kind of interactive communication with his reader. 'Winnicott's writing . . . is surprisingly short on clinical material. This, I believe, is a consequence of the fact that the clinical

Psychoanalytic Thinking in Occupational Therapy: Symbolic, Relational and Transformative, First Edition.
Lindsey Nicholls, Julie Cunningham Piergrossi, Carolina de Sena Gibertoni and Margaret A. Daniel.
© 2013 John Wiley & Sons, Ltd. Published 2013 by John Wiley & Sons, Ltd.

experience is to such a large degree located in the reader's experience of "being read" (that is, of being interpreted, understood) by the writing. When Winnicott does offer clinical material, he often refers not to a specific intervention with a particular patient, but to a "very common experience" in analysis. In this way, he implicitly asks the reader to draw on his own lived experience with patients for the purpose not of "taking in" Winnicott's ideas, but of inviting from the reader an "original response"' (Ogden, 2001, p. 6).

In this chapter the story of Gianni was able to come alive because of how I read Winnicott and how I was read by Winnicott. Telling the story of Gianni's journey with me seemed a fitting way of describing an occupational therapist's 'original response' (as above) to Winnicott's thinking. The chapter will concentrate on the theories of Winnicott concerning what happens in the space of the relationship between therapist and patient. The interesting part for occupational therapists is the presence in the space not only of therapist and patient, but also of activities and 'doing'. My intent is to reflect on how the role of 'doing' using the MOVI (described in Chapter 7) in our therapy sessions becomes much clearer thanks to the thoughts of Donald Winnicott.

Inhabiting the intermediate space

Winnicott is the only psychoanalyst who includes an inanimate object in illustrating his theory about the importance of the first human relationships in human development. For this reason he is particularly interesting for occupational therapists, who include inanimate objects in their therapy sessions and as part of their relationships. He was a paediatrician (Winnicott, 1958) before becoming an analyst and his many contacts with mothers and their young children became a valuable learning area for his future work as a child analyst.

It was in his work as a paediatrician that he became interested in the function of the pieces of cloth, teddy bears and blankets that the children often brought with them during consultations. He called these 'transitional objects' and began to understand them as having the paradoxical function of linking the child to his mother and at the same time providing distance from her. They were further described as 'first possessions' which the child recognised as not being part of himself, 'not-me', and at the same time not a part of his mother (Winnicott, 1971).

This use of an object was important because only by being recognised as not being part of himself (here we are talking about young babies from 4 months to 1 year of age) could the objects become transitional and link the child's inner reality with what was outside of himself (his mother). 'The transitional object is never under magical control like the internal object, nor is it outside control as the real mother is' (Winnicott, 1971, p. 10). The child in this phase of his development is leaving the state of fusion with his mother (characterised by feelings of omnipotence) and beginning to develop a relationship with comings and goings, or losing and finding objects. The fact that the transitional object keeps him connected to his mother but at the same time provides a space for separation from her is an extremely important relational concept in child development and in therapy. The transitional objects exist in a transitional area, also called an intermediate area, which Winnicott (1971) describes as existing between inner reality and outer reality, two parts of human existence to which he adds this third:

> . . . *an intermediate area of* experiencing, *to which inner reality and external life both contribute. It is an area that is not challenged, because no claim is made on its behalf except that it shall exist as a resting-place for the individual engaged in the perpetual human task of keeping inner and outer reality separate yet interrelated.*
>
> (Winnicott, 1971, p. 2)

The intermediate area is a space where creativity is born and where play begins. Winnicott sees creativity and play as fundamental parts of life and as a link between inner and outer reality. For adults he considers cultural experiences such as the arts (painting, poetry or plays) and religion or spirituality as taking place in the space for creativity and play.

Adding doing to the transitional space

In occupational therapy using the Vivaio model (MOVI), as will be seen in Chapter 7, activities and doing are part of the three-way relationship between therapist, patient and doing. They include both real (concrete) and unreal (fantasy, emotional) elements; they link the patient's inner world with outer reality and provide both a closeness to the therapist and at the same time a distance from her (Cunningham Piergrossi, 1992). They clearly possess a transitional function such as that described by Winnicott (1971). But to become truly therapeutic there are many complex aspects which must by taken into consideration, because with disturbed patients it is the therapist's understanding of what is happening that permits the use of the theory itself.

Using the MOVI, we try to create an intermediate space by inviting the patients to choose the materials or activities they are interested in using and to consider how they want to use them. This leads to different kinds of reaction which can range from complete apathy, to refusal, to aggressive destruction. Patients are not always thankful for having choices. In the following considerations about choice I have highlighted aspects particularly pertinent for the case study that will follow.

(1) The possibility of having a free choice of what to do can lead to the illusion of omnipotence. This illusion can be very positive for the patient in the beginning of therapy to have a sense of who he or she is, together with a therapist who remains accepting but firm and sure, but who is not 'destroyed' by the omnipotence. (It is interesting that Winnicott (1971) describes a similar process during adolescence when he writes that parents' most important job in that difficult phase is simply to survive (Chapter 11).) The omnipotent phase in early development is important, according to Winnicott, because it often includes aggressiveness or destruction. The good-enough mother in this phase is completely attuned to the needs of her child as she guides him or her towards maturity. The good-enough therapist is able to accept the feelings of omnipotence in her patient by playing together and respecting the patient's discoveries,

repetitions and grandiosity, and at the same time protecting or emotionally 'holding' them. 'Holding' is a term Winnicott (1971) uses to describe both physical and emotional closeness with young babies.

(2) The materials or actions or sensory experiences chosen by our patients have both an inner and an outer reality. Wood is real wood, and the same is true of paints and flour and eggs and the card game of gin rummy. At the same time there is always an inner experience which is completely subjective. Products can range from bizarre fantasies (considered an object) to wooden objects which can represent an unconscious emotion. Even hate in a game of gin rummy, though conscious, can be considered an inner experience evoked by a real game. All of this happens in a space where the therapist is actively involved in the doing with the patient. 'Psychotherapy takes place in the overlap of two areas of playing, that of the patient and that of the therapist' (Winnicott, 1971, p. 38).

(3) The possibility of choosing also permits the choice of what Winnicott (1971) describes as 'nonsense'. He is referring to what patients want to talk about in psychoanalysis, but in occupational therapy we are referring to what the patient wants to do. Winnicott explains that patients need to be able to free associate, to talk without following a logical sequence or finding a sense to everything they say. The analyst must refrain from immediately looking for sense and connections and making interpretations and stay in the area of creativity and play.

> In the relaxation that belongs to trust and to acceptance of the professional reliability of the therapeutic setting there is room for the idea of unrelated thought sequences which the analyst will do well to accept as such, not assuming the existence of a significant thread.
>
> (Winnicott, 1971, p. 55)

It is tempting as occupational therapists to try to influence the choices of our patients, because we are trained to look at function and to know what is 'best' for them and for their development. But being able to stay with their choices which make no sense to us and play with them can create the relaxation and trust that Winnicott sees as essential in the therapeutic process. This was particularly true in the therapeutic story of Gianni, which is presented below. As Winnicott (1971) stated: 'The individual can come together and exist as a unit, not as a defence against anxiety but as an expression of I AM, I am alive, I am myself. From this position everything is creative' (p. 56).

Gianni at the beginning of his therapy

It was while working with 13-year-old Gianni that I first began to think about occupational therapy sessions as existing in the intermediate space described by Winnicott (1971). It became clear to me at a certain point that the activities we were involved in together served the same function in our relationship as the transitional objects for young children and their mothers, and that our relationship existed in an intermediate space, neither completely real nor completely unreal.

At the beginning of his therapy and for a long time thereafter, Gianni needed what Winnicott calls the illusion of omnipotence, which constitutes the very beginning of the construction of the intermediate space.

> . . . the realm of illusion . . . is at the basis of initiation of experience. . . . made possible by the mother's special capacity for making adaptation to the needs of her infant, thus allowing the infant the illusion that what the infant creates really exists.
>
> (Winnicott, 1971, p. 14)

Learning to play

In spite of his parents' description of a boy without initiative, during therapy Gianni soon showed his feelings of omnipotence as he fashioned himself a king costume, calling himself 'King Break-Everything'. He was the richest and most powerful king in the world as well as being extremely aggressive with the materials in the room. I was able to help him to accept rules, and therefore my presence, only by entering into his king world and adapting to his needs, accepting his delusions, just like a mother does with her infant.

Two examples from those early days: in the first Gianni would go out into the courtyard of the building where our centre is housed and proclaim his power to his people; these were the inhabitants of the apartments facing down into the courtyard. In order to convince him to stay in the therapy room, I wrote a proclamation called 'the king's pact', etched on to a sheet of golden-coloured metal, which we both signed. On the pact was written that King Break-Everything agreed to stay in the room with Julie. In the same period of time he started a book of proclamations written in 'Latin' with a pen with golden ink. There were pages and pages of writing which said nothing. I helped him with these activities by preparing the materials, talking about what the king might be feeling, asking him to give me some 'translations', and trying to make my presence felt and necessary.

This is the perfect example of the 'nonsense' described by Winnicott; an activity that was accepted and shared by Gianni and me. In this phase of omnipotence I was necessary to Gianni as a helper, but not as a real human object to which he could relate; this only came much later. It was as if Gianni were demonstrating a very early phase of relating. In the relationship with his mother, the baby in the phase of the illusion of omnipotence sees her as part of himself. The role of the therapist is not the same as that of the mother, but in establishing a relationship with her patients the phases and their progression can follow a similar pattern to that of an infant and his mother (caregiver). It is often necessary with very disturbed children to encourage and allow their feelings of omnipotence by playing together with them and gradually introducing reality factors. This progression of events was very clear with Gianni.

In that initial part of his therapy he was in constant movement, talking rapidly, using long words disconnected from the real situation or the conversation he was involved in. He was always smiling and cheerful, even when throwing a stool or breaking a piece of wood. He would talk about death, describing macabre accidents without the least expression of emotion. The most disconcerting part of the sessions for the first year of therapy was the anguish we both felt at the end of the hour. The king would melt away before my eyes. Gianni explained that he was reliving the scene in the film *Who Framed Roger Rabbit* (Zemeckis, 1988) when the enemy dissolves in a vat of acid. He would take off his king's robes and decorations one by one, writhing and uttering strangled sounds, ending up lying on the floor completely buried and hidden under the pile of clothes. He would not let me 'save' him or be near to him in any way. After this he would get up and leave the room. I remember talking to him during these moments like a mother talks to a baby, knowing he was not listening to my words but that at least he was hearing my voice.

It may be necessary to explain that Gianni only dressed up as a king during these therapy sessions. In his real life he went to school, had judo lessons, went skiing with his father. He was a tall, good-looking, intelligent boy, with a friendly smile but without any friends except for those procured by his parents. He lived an existence that was extremely linear and rigid, doing everything exactly as his parents told him, and would be completely lost when their instructions did not apply to an unexpected life event. He liked to watch the same videos again and again and would memorise certain facts, such as the dates of birth and death of famous people. In therapy he was a completely different person.

Gianni had been in psychotherapy for several years before coming to occupational therapy and the therapist had interrupted the therapy because of his extreme aggressiveness. In our sessions the presence of the materials and objects in the room permitted a distance from me but at the same time provided a tie to me, just like the young child's transitional object. Dressing as an all-powerful king helped him to feel protected from a relationship with me that was extremely frightening for him, and protected both of us from the aggressiveness he had been unable to control in the 'verbal' (talking only) psychotherapy.

Beginning to play together

For a long time (about a year of twice-weekly sessions) Gianni remained in his fantasy world with me as an ally. He had begun to accept some of my suggestions which were attempts at forming a bridge between unreal and real, and I began to be seen by him as part of the activity and not just as a necessary presence. For example, he finally accepted the idea of writing a book about the king's life instead of the golden penned 'Latin'. In this book he let me be the secretary and he dictated pages and pages of stories of battles and conquests filled with dates. It was very repetitive, and still part of his fantasy as an all-powerful king, but a step towards reality in the sense that we did it together and it was written in a common and real language. He was beginning to let me into his world.

The activity that was probably the most significant in beginning to play together was the printing of dollar bills using the technique of linoleum printing. He designed the bills himself in the different money values, all with the face of the king, each value having a different colour. His aim was to print as many bills as possible and to be the richest king in the world. I remember saying to him one time, 'Wouldn't it be great if all this money were real?' And he answered, 'It is real, and I am the richest king in the world.' The interesting thing about this activity was its anchor to reality. It required careful work, especially in carving the linoleum and then in the printing, using the ink, etc. It wasn't easy for Gianni because, even though he was intelligent and talented artistically, he would become anxious as soon as something simple went wrong, and would drop everything and ask me to finish, saying: 'I abhor making mistakes – you do it,' in his commanding king's voice.

I began to realise that he must have missed out as a young child on all of those trial and error kinds of play, both because of his lack of initiative and because of his parents' taking over too quickly. He needed the reality experience and also to feel the strong emotions that were coming from his inner world, in the presence of a therapist who was ready to help him 'come together and exist as a unit, not as a defence against anxiety but as an expression of I AM, I am alive, I am myself' (Winnicott, 1971, p. 56).

This also meant feeling real emotions, and I remember one Easter vacation, in the last session before the break, he exclaimed in his dramatic way, 'How can I leave my money for such a long time? It hurts too much!' In that moment his money had the clear function of existing in a transitional space between his inner world of illusion and his real world that contained painful separations. It was the first time that I had heard him express the realisation of emotion. Of course, he could not say that he would miss the therapy and myself, but he could express the same thing using the money, his transitional object.

When the production of dollar bills, which he was now completely autonomous in carrying out, became obsessive and seemingly without end, I suggested that we use them for a game that we would invent called 'The King's Life' and he accepted. It was clear to me at this point that he was now ready to accept my interventions that interrupted his obsessive thinking, trusting me and some of my ideas. The King's Life was a kind of Monopoly using dice to go around the board and stopping on various squares where one could either earn or have to pay money according to the instructions, all of which had to do with the king's world and which Gianni helped to invent. It was fun to play with him and to know that for the first time he was accepting a symbolic representation of his fantasy and that he could not control the outcome because it all depended on the throw of the dice. His omnipotence was beginning to waver and to make room for the world of reciprocal interaction. One day he said to me, 'Wouldn't it be great if these dollars were real!'

The end of King Break-Everything

After 3 years of therapy the time had come to try to survive in therapy without the king. I proposed to Gianni that in 6 months' time he could begin to come to our sessions and work on his projects without dressing in the king clothes. He surprised me by accepting rather easily, especially because the 6-month time lapse would give him time to work up gradually to the event itself. We wrote about it, talked about it and began a sort of countdown which he monitored closely. It was during these 6 months, as part of one of his stories about the king, that there was a very touching moment when he pulled a piece of silken cloth from the dressing-up bin and put it around my shoulders, declaring me his queen. He was ready to move on, and when the big day came for the last of the king he simply undressed and I helped him fold up each robe and cape and train with the various crowns and put them all in a box in the cupboard, where they remained for the rest of his therapy, never to be touched or looked at again. We talked often about how the king could now live inside of himself, how he didn't need to dress as a king any more, but of course he could think about him and we could remember him together.

The first activity post-king was a very long series of the card game gin rummy which continued for several months. It represented a decisive entrance to the real world that paradoxically permitted him to communicate another part of his inner world, that of emotion. In the game, which contains a mixture of strategic skill and luck, he could express joy when he won, 'desperation' when he lost, jealousy and hate towards me when I was winning, vendetta when he pulled ahead. He could also laugh together with me at the change of fortune dictated largely by the chance of the cards. I also demonstrated the same kinds of emotion as he did and was amazed at the relational capacities of Gianni, which I had never seen before. It is interesting to note here that I cannot remember who chose the game of gin rummy, which brings to mind a concept that Winnicott (1971) emphasises repeatedly in his writing about the beginning of the transitional object. 'Of the transitional object it can be said that it is a matter of agreement between us and the baby that we will never ask the question: "Did you conceive of this or was it presented to you from without?" The important point is that no decision on this point is expected' (p. 12)

The real world

Gianni remained a youth of few words. It was very difficult to carry on a conversation with him because he would answer questions with standard, everyday phrases or repeat back to me what I had just said. For this reason his involvement in activities was extremely important. He enjoyed cooking and cooked the same cake recipe for several months. It was a complicated process because it involved dividing the yolk from the white and whipping the white. It took him many trials to succeed, and when he failed he would again ask me to take over. I remember the day he succeeded in dividing the egg perfectly. He looked at me in amazement and said, 'It's a miracle!' 'No, Gianni,' said I. 'It wasn't a miracle; it was you. You worked at it, you learned and you did it.' Thinking about this episode and many other similar situations, I could almost imagine Gianni floating above reality, every once in a while touching down, but remaining surprised at what he found, sometimes disconcerted and sometimes pleased.

I think it was by inhabiting the intermediate space that he was able to begin to spend more time and mental space in the real world. This was probably because in the intermediate space he had begun to really see himself. Winnicott (1971) might say that he was shedding his 'false self' (p. 102). The activities in this phase of his therapy were all reality oriented. He did invent stories and paint and draw interesting and elaborate works of art, but they were all representations of his inner world and he recognised them as such, producing real paintings and written stories.

On the home front he finished a high school for graphic design and began an apprentice job for a design company, helped by the school. He started out fine, but then began to have serious problems paying attention at work, following instructions, understanding his mistakes. For example, one of his assignments was to count a certain number of pages to put together in a particular way for a shipment. This was an easy job for an intelligent boy like Gianni, but each pile ended up with a different number of pages every time and his boss couldn't understand why he wasn't able to learn from his mistakes. One day he was asked to stay for overtime to help finish an important job and without saying anything he picked up his jacket and left. Gianni had a schedule in his head which gave him structure and security, and in this case included the bus ride with his favourite bus driver, who had become his friend. He would have missed the bus if he had stayed later at work. Needless to say, that was the end of his job in a real-life company.

This was Gianni. During this period he was more pensive and less jolly during therapy and began to draw what was happening at work. (He would tell me that everything was fine there, no problems.) In his drawings he was surrounded by boxes and stacks of papers and was always alone. In one of these drawings, he drew a line down the middle of the page and put himself on one side, seated at his table with a computer, and on the other side he drew strange wiggly marks, stars and scribbles, and he explained to me that those were his thoughts, and that when they entered his head he could no longer concentrate on his work.

There followed a long period where he and his parents came to terms with the necessity of declaring his invalidity in order to have a special work placement for him. It was a difficult time for them, and they were helped very much by a psychotherapist who enabled them to see Gianni as he really was, without needing any more to create the Gianni of their desires. It was during these months that he was able to pass his driving exam and came to his therapy sessions driving the car.

Gianni's words towards the end of his therapy gave voice to his confused thoughts as he became more reflective and able to be more in contact with the real world around him. 'I feel like I don't experience emotions fully. I feel them, but it's as if something were missing,' he said with one of his big smiles. I told him that his words had moved me greatly, and he became more pensive. I added, talking about our long therapeutic journey together, that the emotions are there, they are not lacking, but they seem to be buried or ignored because they are frightening, and he listened, thought about it and agreed.

One day he said, without any prompting from me, 'You helped me to go towards the future.' This was the same boy who at the beginning of his therapy had said that he only wanted to live in the past.

Conclusions

When I am in the intermediate space with a patient, I feel like I can be myself and he can be himself, or in other words my play is interspersed with his and both of us are free to be creative. I feel like I can really take in what he brings to the space and try to use it creatively, without judging or trying to change or feeling attacked. In the intermediate space I am free from theories, from techniques, from knowing what to do, and can 'be' as a therapist. I feel protected and concentrate completely on the present moment. All of this might seem easy, but this is far from true. As we have seen with Gianni's story, it took a long time to really be able to be together with him.

Maybe the most important of Winnicott's lessons is that the good-enough mother knows how to be with her baby, how to adapt to his needs. The good-enough therapist, by the same verse, knows how to be with her patient and to adapt to his needs while maintaining her adultness and using her own creativity to enable that of her patient. Winnicott did not teach us techniques; he taught us to 'be with', to 'listen to', to 'believe in'. When we work, we don't think about theory; we think about what is happening between ourselves, our patient and the activity we are engaged in. It is very interesting, however, to see how our work seems to fit in so well with the intuition and ideas of great thinkers like Winnicott. This is because therapy necessarily follows the path of development, and a patient who develops his own sense of self becomes creative and responsible for his own life. Then what happens is all up to him; our part is done.

I hope it has been clear to the reader that in my work with Gianni I was always aware of two things: one, that his path necessarily included understanding the difference between real and not real; and two, that he was working on having an idea of who he was as a person in his own right, constructing a self not dictated by anyone else. My job was to help him in these two very difficult tasks, especially difficult because he had not managed to come to terms with them earlier in his life and had constructed all kinds of defences that did not permit him to accept help from anyone. So the therapist's task is not simply to follow the trail of normal development, because the patient does not allow it. The therapist must use her own creativity to coax very frightened patients like Gianni back into the world of relationships and emotions, with all the problems, difficulties and potential joy that this new maturity can bring.

References

Cunningham Piergrossi, J. (1992) Il reale. *Il Ruolo Terapeutico (rubrica Vivaio)*, 59, 50–52.

Milne, A. A. (1927) *Now We Are Six*. New York: Dell.

Ogden, T. (2001) Reading Winnicott. *Psychoanalytic Quarterly*, 70 (2), 299–324.

Winnicott, D. W. (1958) *Through Paediatrics to Psychoanalysis*. London: Karnac, 1992.

Winnicott, D. W. (1971) *Playing and Reality*. New York: Basic Books.

Zemeckis, R. L. (1988) *Who Framed Roger Rabbit* (dir. R. L. Zemeckis), Touchstone Pictures, California.

5 Beyond Bowlby: Exploring the Dynamics of Attachment

Margaret Daniel

This chapter goes beyond Bowlby and Ainsworth's ground-breaking work on attachment theory to give an overview of how the contemporary relational theory of attachment has been extended into the field of adult attachment. Through the inspired work of Dorothy Heard and Brian Lake (1997) and in collaboration with Una McCluskey's (2005) observational research work, this chapter will introduce the interpersonal process of attachment based explorative interest sharing. This theory is a new approach to thinking about the self, through creating a dynamic restorative process, which Heard and Lake call the Theory of Attachment Based Explorative Interest Sharing (TABEIS). Informed by their work, McCluskey (2011a) has gradually, over the last decade, developed a new model of practice called Exploratory Goal Corrected Psychotherapy (EGCP)©. For health care professionals such as occupational therapists, the approach can assist the practitioner to bridge the distance between people through developing a more vital and creative approach in their use of activity to promote recovery and restore well-being (Scottish Government, 2010).

Introduction

How do our early experiences shape our lives? From our very beginnings we are programmed to be relational creatures, striving to seek out someone who will help us to survive by making us feel safe and secure. From our earliest moments of existence we are attached within the safety of our mother's womb. To understand more about the self as a whole, we need to take account of the emotional environment in which we reside (Gerhardt, 2010). Within the caregiving environment of the occupational therapy profession, people are encouraged to become involved in activities that are designed to have a restorative quality, under the belief that creative activity is beneficial to a person's health and well-being

Psychoanalytic Thinking in Occupational Therapy: Symbolic, Relational and Transformative, First Edition.
Lindsey Nicholls, Julie Cunningham Piergrossi, Carolina de Sena Gibertoni and Margaret A. Daniel.
© 2013 John Wiley & Sons, Ltd. Published 2013 by John Wiley & Sons, Ltd.

(Griffiths, 2008). Yet as the researcher Reynolds (2000) highlights, the links between creative interests and well-being are mostly implied. The occupational therapists Timmons and MacDonald (2008) have noted that, although creative activities have a positive effect on health and enhance psychological well-being, it is not clear how this comes about. From an academic perspective, Sadlo (2004) would consider that the profession could benefit from an increased awareness of other sciences.

The innovative work of TABEIS has grown out of the additional psychoanalytic knowledge beyond Freud, influenced by object relations thinking through Guntrip, Winnicott and Fairbairn. This new model of self is a work in progress and is continuing to be shaped and formed by material gleaned from Una McCluskey's extensive research data gathered from her work with professional caregivers (Heard, Lake and McCluskey, 2009; Heard, McCluskey and Lake, 2011; McCluskey, 2010, 2011a, 2011b).

Beginning with Bowlby

The British child psychiatrist and psychoanalyst John Bowlby (1907–1990) has always challenged the psychoanalytic world with his influential 'attachment theory', showing how the quality of our early relationships has an impact upon the effectiveness of our occupational activities through the choices we make. Bowlby had great respect for the scientific approach Sigmund Freud applied to his early clinical observations, but Freud maintained his view of objects (human, artefact or ideas) as instinctual and intrapersonal, which Bowlby regarded as only part of the picture. He believed the relationship also required an interpersonal engagement with a person or object. Bowlby considered his research went some way towards raising the status of psychoanalysis to a science by evidencing and improving the approach. However, his ideas were perceived by some of the psychoanalytic world as not being psychoanalytic enough, due to his interest in the close relational bonds that support exploration and self-development (Lemma, 2003; Hinde, 2005).

Bowlby's observations originally had more influence on research and social policy than on clinical practice. He believed that the child's unique relational environment had a huge impact upon their internal environment, and influenced the growing person's actions and choices throughout their life. Currently his ideas are growing in popularity as emphasis on evidence-based practice gives an opportunity to build on his thinking (Fonagy and Target, 2003).

John Bowlby came from a psychoanalytic background and aligned himself with the less inward-looking Object Relations School of thinking. He considered that central to a person's psychological well-being are the important emotional bonds that get established with others, especially in childhood with the first adult caregiver (usually the mother). His interest in attachment grew from the year he spent as a volunteer working with disturbed children, made homeless at the end of the Second World War (Grossman, Grossman and Waters, 2005); a time which Jeremy Holmes (1996), the eminent psychotherapist, believed had a detrimental effect on child development. Added to this was Bowlby's own personal experience of distant parenting, which may have further influenced his curiosity about the child's relational experiences with their parents (Shilkret and Shilkret, 2008).

In his early twenties, Bowlby was asked to write a report for the World Health Organisation and in it he highlighted that the foundations to a child's well-being was 'a warm, intimate and continuous relationship with his mother (or permanent mother-substitute)' (Bowlby, 1969/82, pp. xi–xii; quoted in Heard, Lake and Mc-Cluskey, 2009/11, p. 225). The special relationship a child forms with his or her closest caregiver is attachment and can be either secure (reliable) or insecure (unpredictable) (Shemilt and Naismith, 2006). Influential to Bowlby's thinking were James and Joyce Robertson (1952), who captured on film the distressing impact of young children being separated (briefly and longer term) from their parents through admission to hospital or attendance at a residential nursery. The films powerfully illustrate the emotional trauma of being deprived of a mother's affection and security, and have been influential in shaping present health and day care practices. Based on their experiences, they highlighted three ways a child could respond to their mother's absence, by *protesting*, *withdrawing* or *detaching* from the situation (Bowlby, 1969/82, 1973, p. 35). From this, they were able to illustrate how important it was to have regular and reliable contact with an attachment figure, who could intuitively attend to a child's careseeking needs (Fonagy and Target, 2003).

Bowlby discovered that the key to attachment theory was the melding of developmental psychology with open systems theory through the new field of ethology, which studied animal behaviour and gave his work a secure scientific base. He believed that primitive animal behaviour patterns could help shed light on the normal process of human attachment. For some, this biological focus was viewed as a shift away from his psychoanalytic roots and, of course, it was not without its controversy as it touched on the sensitive subject of parents' caregiving skills (Holmes, 1993; Gomez, 1997).

Bowlby's focus was on the interplay between the two instinctive systems of careseeking and caregiving, in which a child (careseeker) at play becomes distressed, and will go in search of a parent or parent figure (caregiver) who will comfort and soothe them so that they can return to their play. Bowlby's interest was drawn to the baby's need to have an empathic caregiver, who could alter his or her behaviour in order to satisfy the careseeker's goal of survival (the process of goal-corrected empathic attunement observed and described by McCluskey (2005)). Once the goals of careseeking and caregiving are met, both systems become inactive (goal-corrected), but if this is not achieved then both people will continue to feel deeply distressed (see McCluskey, 2005).

The intensity of Bowlby's vision concentrated on measuring the changes in closeness between the careseeker and caregiver. However, he failed to notice the nature of the interaction that led to the state of well-being in the careseeking child, which in turn enabled the child to return to what they were previously doing. As I will discuss later, Heard and Lake (Heard and Lake, 1997; Heard, Lake and McCluskey, 2009; Heard, McCluskey and Lake, 2011) subsequently focused on the quality of this caregiving, believing that the relationship was a dynamic process, important for survival, as well as restoring the child's exploratory capacity and sense of well-being.

To maintain well-being throughout our daily lives we require more than Bowlby's two instinctive goal-corrected systems of attachment – careseeking and caregiving. People are sociable creatures and make attachments to others, especially in infancy, which increases a child's chances of survival. Moreover, these attachments form an internal virtual database. Bowlby called this the 'internal working model', which continues to influence and inform our everyday actions throughout our lives (Holmes, 1994). Our earliest relational moments become the templates that are encased within our minds and shape our future emotional development and ethical values, imprinted within our neural pathways even before words have been formed (Balbernie, 2001; Gerhardt, 2010).

Alongside Bowlby in pioneering attachment theory was the American psychologist Mary Ainsworth. She provided the empirical evidence through her observational work of mother/infant interactions in their natural surroundings in Uganda and by developing, with her colleagues, the Strange Situation Test in the United Kingdom (Shilkret and Shilkret, 2008). The Strange Situation Test (Ainsworth, Blehar, Waters and Walls, 1978) is an observational procedure that highlights the importance of a child's reaction when separated from their mother or primary caregiver, and more importantly the child's response on her return (Bretherton, 2005). Children who have *secure* attachments to their mothers will initially get upset and protest at her absence, but on her return will be able to accept her reassurance and return to their exploratory play.

Insecure attachments can evoke three forms of responses. A child with *insecure avoidant* (deactivating) attachment will carry on as if mother is not there when she returns. A child with *insecure ambivalent* (hyperactivating) attachment gets fussed over and gives mother a hard time, resisting her attempts to soothe, and is unable to be settled (Holmes, 2010). An *insecure disorganised* attachment is seen in a few children and was perplexing for the researchers to categorise, as their behaviour was not always consistent. They may freeze or collapse or head-bang, and were later given a further classification of *disorganised/avoidant* (Bowlby, 1988, p. 125).

To extend the idea of attachment for adults, a student of Mary Ainsworth's, Mary Main, and her research colleagues, developed a tool for measuring adult attachment styles called the Adult Attachment Interview (AAI), in which retrospective childhood memories of attachment experiences were elicited. This classified adults into: *Secure/Autonomous*, *Insecure/Dismissing*, *Insecure/Preoccupied* or *Unresolved* (Fonagy and Target, 2003, p. 239).

Towards well-being

It was the psychotherapist Dorothy Heard (Heard and Lake, 1986) who recognised the importance of Mary Ainsworth's data and saw the core of our attachment dynamic as rooted in our social relationships with others. When Heard (Heard, 1978; Heard and Lake, 1986) met with Ainsworth, she astutely noticed a close similarity between Ainsworth's notion of exploration and Winnicott's (1971, p. 47) concept of 'play', although they were from different theoretical backgrounds

(Heard, Lake and McCluskey, 2009; Heard, McCluskey and Lake, 2011). Dorothy Heard trained in child psychiatry within John Bowlby's department at the Tavistock Clinic and considered that there was a strong relationship between the child's ability to explore and the nature of the caregiver's input. Both, she considered, were restorative, bringing back playfulness to the child once reunited and responded to by their mother in a calming manner (McCluskey, 2005). In partnership with Brian Lake (1986), Dorothy Heard (Heard, Lake and McCluskey, 2009; Heard, McCluskey and Lake, 2011) extended and modified these concepts for adults, to include a new way of organising the self through seven integrated biological systems, which they call 'The Restorative Process':

- Careseeking
- Caregiving
- Exploratory Interest Sharing
- Affectionate Sexuality
- Self-defence
- Internal Supportive/Unsupportive System
- External Supportive/Unsupportive System

In 2009, Heard and Lake incorporated the fear system into their conceptualisation of the restorative process. They did this by locating the older system of fear within the system for self-defence. The fear system is essential as it keeps us alive and safe. When facing circumstances that induce fear, we operate out of our fear system (to get us out of danger) and our attachment/careseeking system (to find someone who will look after us) as well as our internal and external supportive/unsupportive systems, which can either support us or let us down. While this is happening we are unable to caregive and our exploratory interest sharing and affectionate sexuality are lowered considerably (Heard, Lake and McCluskey, 2009; Heard, McCluskey and Lake, 2011). This chapter will go on to describe how a person can operate between Heard and Lake's seven biological systems, which interact with each other as part of the dynamic process to restore well-being in the self.

From her growing research base, Una McCluskey would consider that if we are working therapeutically then 'an understanding of the dynamics of attachment and interest sharing in adult life are essential' (2011b, p. 12). She developed Ainsworth's studies on caregiving responses through her own research, which examined the adult careseeker's exploratory capacity when responded to in different ways by professional caregivers.

In collaboration with Dorothy Heard (Brian Lake died in the winter of 2007), McCluskey continues to refine their ideas on attachment dynamics based on the wealth of material she has collated from professional caregivers, who have been examining their own restorative processes in experiential groups across Britain and Ireland (McCluskey, 2008, 2010, 2011a, 2011b; Heard, Lake and McCluskey, 2009; Heard, McCluskey and Lake, 2011).

Table 5.1 outlines my understanding of the functions and goals of the different systems within Heard and Lake's new conceptualisation of the self (Heard, Lake and McCluskey, 2009; Heard, McCluskey and Lake, 2011).

Table 5.1   The attachment system's function and goals

Attachment system	Function	Goal
Careseeking	Following a threat to the self, to seek help and influence a caregiver to respond	To have the careseeking needs met
Caregiving	1. Protect careseeker from danger, soothe and regulate 2. Inform and respond to careseeker's interests and help forward plan and move into world of peers	To restore the careseeker's well-being and competence by attending to their needs
Exploratory Interest Sharing	Engage in mutually enjoyable interests, alongside likeminded peers, exploring in a supportive companionable way	To experience increased well-being and creativity with intensified vitality, increased confidence and satisfaction
Affectionate Sexuality	To form a secure and enduring intimate relationship with intensified affection which may lead to reproduction	To have heightened pleasure and vitality
Self-defence	1. To protect and keep you alive and out of danger without additional help 2. To search out a caregiver who will protect 3. Aided by the additional help from the two systems below	To survive with well-being
Internal Environment Supportive/Unsupportive System	To help manage threats to well-being, especially when alone, through staying connected to recollections of previous supportive interactions	The only system not goal corrected – it is activated by reminders in the 'here and now' and has an intrapersonal goal
External Environment Supportive/Unsupportive System	To self-create and maintain a way of life 1. With maximum well-being 2. In pleasurable surroundings 3. With a spiritual quality	To achieve sensory satisfaction from one's lifestyle which has an intrapersonal goal

Careseeking

When an infant feels under threat, their fear level soars and arouses their careseeking system, which remains activated until a caregiver (usually the mother or close family member) is located. If the caregiver is able to settle the careseeker's distress, by being appropriately responsive (attuned), they will have successfully assisted the careseeker to achieve their goal by settling their fear and providing encouragement to go on exploring. These two systems operate at an unconscious level and are different, but complementary, goal-corrected systems: that is, they stop once the careseeking goal is reached, only to become aroused again when another threat is sensed and an attentive caregiver is required (McCluskey, 2005). Until then the mother becomes the secure base from which the child can explore. All these interactions, whether they are positive or negative, become stored in what Heard and Lake (Heard, Lake and McCluskey, 2009, p. 117) call our 'internal supportive or unsupportive system' and unconsciously influence the outcome of later encounters. As adults we may be more alert to situations that arouse our fears and have appropriate defences.

Caregiving

A caregiver's system gets aroused when a careseeker approaches them for help and two types of caregiving can be exhibited. The first directly assists the careseeker in an empathic way and has a protective function which settles and calms the careseeker's heightened state of arousal by what the researcher Daniel Stern (1985, p. 145) would call 'purposeful misattunement' – the brief moments when a mother can alter the baby's emotional state by slightly adjusting her pitch, tone of voice or facial expression to let the baby know they are on the same wavelength. A caregiving approach needs to be rapid and sensitive to the infant's emotional needs (Gerhardt, 2004).

The second form of caregiving that Heard and Lake (1986, p. 79) describe has a more 'educative interest sharing component' that can let us forward plan and help in the transition of reliance from parents to peers. This form of caregiving comes after the first and we need to be able to move subtly between the two forms, which some people are unable to manage. In this communicating process, professional caregivers all have patterns of effective and ineffective caregiving, which need to be monitored, alongside being in touch with the wide range of emotions that careseeking can evoke. If a therapist is driven by fear to respond, they will be operating from a defensive caregiving position, which will keep them at a distance from their clients/patients. McCluskey (2005) considers that effective caregiving drives the whole attachment dynamic.

Exploratory interest sharing

Unlike careseeking, which is activated at birth, the interest-sharing system starts around the age of 3 with the rudimentary sharing of activities with playmates. Up until this point, parents have been encouraging interests and rehearsing these skills by joining them in play as 'potential peers' (Heard, Lake and McCluskey, 2009, p. 75). Infants are curious about each other at this time and play alongside one another. Mutual play develops by 4 years, when children have an awareness of another person's viewpoint. However, this still requires adult supervision up until about the age of 6 years, which helps to regulate a child's fear if it has been triggered. Mastery is not achieved until our mid-twenties and requires to be fine-tuned throughout our lives. But if we have not had enough effective caregiving then our sense of security will not enable us to interest share. When the infant feels secure, they are able to explore (Heard, Lake and McCluskey, 2009; Heard, McCluskey and Lake, 2011).

Again, the way we activate our interests is different from the other systems as it will be influenced by what we were told and encouraged to do as children and whether we were guided towards likeminded companions. Interests are the things that absorb us, and what we feel passionate about. They can be explored individually by activities such as engaging in art, writing poetry or playing a musical instrument. Interests also have the potential to be shared, in pairs or groups, with people who have similarly matched interests but do not need to be of similar age. Being with others who share our interests can have an uplifting effect – to boost confidence, validate and affirm. Sharing our interests is something that can be done without empathy, but for a group to reach its longer-term goals requires an empathic member to gel the group together (Heard and Lake, 1997; Heard, Lake and McCluskey, 2009; Heard, McCluskey and Lake, 2011).

Interest sharing has an interpersonal goal and can be either explorative or non-explorative. Working exploratively within this system will mean a person can reach new creative insights ('Eureka' moments) and deepen their understanding, developing skills and enhancing their techniques through observing others performing a similar activity. Heard and Lake note that this will result in restoring a person's well-being with 'new vitality' and 'validation' from those around them who appreciate their achievement (Heard, Lake and McCluskey, 2009, p. 95). Creativity does not have to be exceptional and can include new ideas or activities that have a hint of originality. Sharing these ideas with others can then fuel our passion to create something we could not have done on our own.

If, however, as a child we were prematurely pulled out of our interest sharing to caregive for an adult who was sick, or stand in for a parent who had died, it activates the attachment/caregiving system, which in turn may override our interest-sharing system and prevent us from being explorative. I invite you, as an adult reader of this chapter, to consider who took an interest in you. Did they encourage you to develop interests? Did they help you to find your peers? Did they encourage you to return to your interest when other aspects of life got in the way? Could you return to your interests in a supportive way? Were you given the right materials and put in touch with others who shared these interests with you in an explorative and creative way (McCluskey, 2011b)?

We also can experience a non-explorative form of interest sharing in the passing on of known information and this can be *constructive* (sharing familiar information) or *destructive* (spiteful gossiping). It can be helpful in attempting to get closer to people, and we can also use laughter and humour as short-term ways of achieving intimacy. This type of interest sharing works to achieve a response from a caregiver, but is not a 'Eureka' moment, as experienced in exploratory interest sharing, where more knowledge is learnt. Nevertheless, for those securely attached it can be useful, and it can be essential for those who are insecurely attached to have a way to engage with their caregivers and have a better balance to their well-being. But this is at the cost of maintaining a more distant defensive stance (Heard, Lake and McCluskey, 2009; Heard, McCluskey and Lake, 2011).

The case example will illustrate the concept of exploratory interest sharing through the story of Ruth, who was attending an occupational therapy group at her local resource centre.

Ruth's butterflies

Ruth had arrived at her weekly session and was noticeably upset. She explained to the occupational therapist (OT) that her friend's mother had just died following a long illness, and that she and her friend had been talking late into the night about her life. One of the things her friend's mother had always wanted to experience was to be with the butterflies, to be with nature, and she had organised a humanist funeral for herself so that she could be buried in a wicker coffin in a designated forest.

Ruth wanted to do something for her friend to mark this event. As she spoke and felt listened to by the therapist, her distress began to settle. She felt more present in the room and chose to make something from the material available, some dyed glassine paper, wire and a couple of pipe cleaners. She carried on talking and in that moment it just seemed that she knew what she wanted to do. Influenced by an earlier interest in art, Ruth latched on to an old idea and picked up a magazine, searching for pictures of butterflies. She then cut the papers in the shape of the butterflies, bent the wire, added the pipe cleaners and all of a sudden the materials came alive. They seemed to take on a different form as they gently moved back and forth in the air. Excited by her achievement Ruth packed 12 of them into a shoebox and took them away with her at the end of the session (see Figures 5.1 and 5.2).

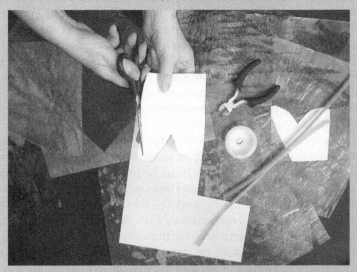

Figure 5.1   Construction of the butterflies. Photograph taken by M. Daniel.

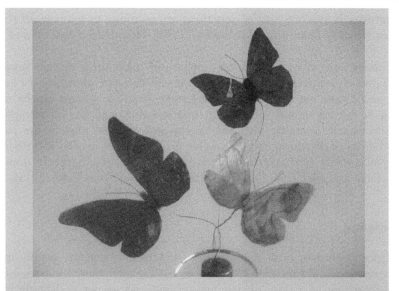

Figure 5.2   Fluttering butterflies. Photograph taken by M. Daniel.

The OT heard later that they had actually been attached to the wicker coffin, and as it was carried the butterflies seemed to float and fly round the coffin in a very magical way that her friend greatly appreciated. It really seemed to have made its mark for Ruth as she achieved a real sense of validation in having been able to offer something to this occasion that was personal and inspiring.

Affectionate sexuality

This is the least understood of the systems, which Heard and Lake (1997) acknowledge in their book *The Challenge of Attachment for Caregiving*. Involved in the affectionate sexual system are pleasurable feelings, raised vitality and the forming of enduring intimate relationships.

The system tracks a similar route to interest sharing, as it can grow out of friendships where people are drawn to sharing and exploring interests together. Someone who is passionate about their interests can attract others to them and their excitement can arouse sexual feelings when a couple are caught up in this heightened state. Heard and Lake (Heard and Lake, 1997; Heard, Lake and McCluskey, 2009; Heard, McCluskey and Lake, 2011) resist calling it 'love', as it lacks a clear translation.

Our sexual feelings surface developmentally when we go through puberty, as we are bombarded with hormones that alter our physical appearance, taking us out of childhood and into adolescence. Although able to be sexually active, adolescents lack control over their emotional arousal, which does not develop until maturity is reached and is something we continue to manage all through our lives (Heard, Lake and McCluskey, 2009; Heard, McCluskey and Lake, 2011).

Affectionate sexuality operates to deepen and maintain a mutual supportive intimacy, which is interpersonal in its goal. It will be active alongside the interest-sharing and caregiving systems. In its defensive form the system can be used in isolation to distract or self-soothe (e.g. masturbation) and has an intrapersonal goal. Affectionate sexuality also has an essential part to play in the parental responsibilities of creating a child through reproduction. However, as with interest sharing, when fear is triggered our affectionate sexuality markedly diminishes (Heard, Lake and McCluskey, 2009; Heard, McCluskey and Lake, 2011).

Self-defence

Self-defence comprises both the fear and attachment systems, which are two separate systems, and functions to return well-being after there has been a threat. Our emotions are in a state of dynamic tension and we are constantly moving between these systems to try to achieve an aspired state of well-being (McCluskey, 2010).

A person's fear system is triggered by something that has been perceived as a hazard and, according to LeDoux (1998), operates to help a person to survive dangerous situations through taking alternative action (flight), standing their ground and taking direct action (fight), or halting the activity (freeze). These responses are out of our awareness but can be useful defences that get us out of danger. When afraid we can either dominate or control another person, but if they are too strong, we shift into appeasing and submitting to their wishes (dominant/submissive).

Through the utilisation of the careseeking system, our personal defence mechanism gives us adaptable ways of operating (unconscious) to keep our fear at bay and avoid the fears generated from our youth (Gerhardt, 2004). Few of us have a robust self-defence system and there will be times when we are overwhelmed by fear or find it hard to think and lose sight of our original task. McCluskey (2010, personal communication) views TABEIS work as 'learning to sustain empathy in the face of fear'.

Internal and External Supportive and Unsupportive Systems

Heard and Lake (Heard and Lake, 1997; Heard, Lake and McCluskey, 2009; Heard, McCluskey and Lake, 2011) realised the importance of Bowlby's (1969/82) Internal Working Model (IWM) and added a further two systems to support the other five systems in the restorative process. These are the *Internal Supportive/Unsupportive* and *External Supportive/Unsupportive Systems*, which function through the IWM to offer support and assistance to a person when his/her well-being has been threatened, and especially at points when there is no one around to help. Unlike the other systems, these internal and external environments are intrapersonal, in that they are reached from within the person themselves.

Being made to feel welcomed and wanted is fundamental to who we are, and if we are parented in a supportive way, right from our entry into the world, then this will influence who we become and etch in our minds a sense of self. At points of threat when we are on our own, we need to rely on giving the support to ourselves through the stored inner resources of past encounters or by actively finding someone to give us the support, as we require. However, if a lot of our relational experiences were unsupportive and our needs went unmet, then our inner repertoire of supportive figures may be somewhat depleted. Likewise, if our environment is filled with dominating and controlling figures (or worse) rather than supportive and companionable ones, then our internal environment will also reflect this. We will lack the motivation to seek someone out, as we may anticipate being let down. This leaves us with an internal system that feels unsupportive, unsafe and overwhelmed by fear.

The Internal Supportive/Unsupportive System

The internal environment is a system that is not goal corrected and keeps in touch with the IWM to influence and revise who we think we are (Heard, Lake and McCluskey, 2009; Heard, McCluskey and Lake, 2011). If we have enough *supportive* experiences, like a teacher affirming our work or an aunt warmly encouraging our achievements, then these experiences will be influential in influencing future encounters. However, if the responses were *unsupportive* (e.g. if we were repeatedly told that we were hopeless or stupid), then this can create assumptions that will colour and distort our view of the external environment, making us cautious of others and unable to trust. Hence our internal and external environments are shaped by our relational experiences, which inform the choices we make.

As therapists, it would therefore seem important to have an awareness of the IWM and how it influences not only the client/patient, but the therapist's own internal and external environments in a supportive or unsupportive way, as this can either help or hinder their interactions. Our internal supportive/unsupportive system is the core of who we are and it is useful to note that our minds have the potential to exchange or replace older models (Heard, Lake and McCluskey, 2009; Heard, McCluskey and Lake, 2011).

The External Supportive/Unsupportive System

Heard and Lake (1986, 1997) would consider our external supportive system to be the lifestyle that we create from the warmly remembered childhood places where we felt at our most secure and explorative. This external environment influences the way we shape our surroundings, by creating a setting that comes from our inner imaginings (intrapersonal goal), informed by our past familiar surroundings and limited by the constraints of our intellect and financial income. It can allow us to feel 'at home' with what we construct, include, and do, within this self-created space. However, if we share our living space with a partner, who does not share the same tastes and interests as ourselves, we may have to negotiate and come to some sort of compromise. At points, this system can be constructed defensively and maintained by the unsupportive internal system, which may have previously experienced an external environment that was disruptive, through domestic violence, marital breakdown, damage to property, or financial worries (Heard, Lake and McCluskey, 2009; Heard, McCluskey and Lake, 2011).

At times we all need to move back into an area of subjectivity and the internal and external environments of these supportive/unsupportive systems can be used when we are alone as memory reminders that are activated to help us cope with any threats to our well-being, which may arise when there is no one available (Heard, Lake and McCluskey, 2009; Heard, McCluskey and Lake, 2011). I will now go on to examine how this dynamic restorative process can assist a therapist to be better informed about themselves and their clinical practice.

Restoring occupational well-being

The structure of health care within mental health continues to evolve and in their informative textbook Atkinson and Wells (2000) suggest there has been a shift towards a collaborative 'doing with' approach that emphasises the relational nature of the process. Sadlo (2004) believes that therapists require the ability to collaborate with individuals, using not only their professional skills and knowledge, but also their own creativity. As Timmons and MacDonald (2008) have noted, there is uncertainty as to how the positive effect on health and well-being comes about, while Holder (2001) would consider that activity is a necessary component of well-being.

A recent feature in the *OTNews* by Anita Holford (2011) again draws attention to the benefits of creative activity in maintaining an individual's health and well-being, noting that the UK government's project entitled '5 Ways to Wellbeing' (Nef, 2008) encourages us to build relationships with others by making space to become actively involved in new and challenging ways that continue to build on learning in a sharing and supportive way. I believe this fits with Heard, Lake and McCluskey's (Heard, Lake and McCluskey, 2009; Heard, McCluskey and Lake, 2011) view of the importance of understanding the dynamics of attachment and exploratory interest sharing. In addition, McCluskey (2011b, p. 14) emphasises that 'access to an effective caregiver is central to the wellbeing of a person throughout the whole of their lives'. It would seem to me that Heard and Lake's (Heard, Lake and McCluskey, 2009; Heard, McCluskey and Lake, 2011) new paradigm is a possible guide that can assist occupational therapists and other professional caregivers to restore well-being dynamically through an understanding of how the attachment system operates.

As caregiving professionals, occupational therapists need to be able to utilise their capacity to be creative by having an awareness of how activity is influenced by the fear and attachment systems. Dorothy Heard would advise that we take account of a person's creative interests, which may have become 'frozen' or still lie undiscovered (Heard, Lake and McCluskey, 2009, p. 48). Therapy may provide an opportunity to 'defrost' the past interests, and enable the activities to be reformed to fit with the person's current lifestyle. Endorsing this idea, Schmid (2005), an occupational therapy lecturer from Australia who has worked within the field of mental health, emphasises in her rich textbook on creativity the lifelong importance of maintaining creative interests.

Kirstie's choice

Kirstie was attending the occupational therapy department following her recent admission to the acute admission ward. While she was looking at some of the activities she could choose, a silk painting kit caught her attention and she asked the therapist if she could try it out. Instead of agreeing, the therapist began to distract Kirstie away from the kit and on to some clay which had already been opened and was able to be used immediately. Kirstie nodded and began to work with the clay. The experienced therapist was surprised by her own response to the situation and brought this event to supervision, where she described how she had begun to distract Kirstie, filling the space with light chat so as to lower her own growing sense of discomfort. The therapist was able to see that her fear had grown when the silk painting activity had been suggested. She could only think about her own fear at never having used this activity before.

The therapist knew that she did not want to be seen as incompetent and reacted by busying up, filling the space with nervous talk that took Kirstie's attention away from her chosen activity. From a TABEIS perspective, the therapist had moved into a defensive position in which she was no longer able to be in an effective caregiving role, as her own fear system had been triggered. In supervision she was able to recognise that her own early experiences around 'getting it right' had aroused a memory that left her feeling she had to 'get it right' in the session.

Kirstie, too, will have been anxious about being in a new situation and operating out of her own fear system, similar to the therapist. If the therapist had been monitoring her own body responses, she would have picked up that her fear system had been aroused and been able to regulate it, by centring first herself and then Kirstie. They may then have been able to explore the new activity together, shifting the relationship into one less about control (dominant/submissive) and more about supportive collaboration (supportive companionable) where new learning could have been discovered together, returning a sense of competence and well-being to them both.

At points of ill-health, when a person is often caught up in seeking care, the fear system is aroused and will disrupt the dynamic balance of exploration and creativity. The American occupational therapist Mary Reilly (1974) was developing the idea of the work/play balance and suggested that individuals are driven by their curiosity to be explorative. As Thomson and Blair (1998) propose, creative activity could be considered a reasonable form of play for adults. It requires a safe enough environment, where fear is at a minimum, so that risk can be attempted in the pioneering steps beyond the familiar routine, venturing into moments of new discovery. Schmid (2005) importantly notes that this pursuit also requires to be shared with our peers, so that a person's achievements can be validated. For this to happen, Heard and Lake (1997) suggest, we need to move out of a careseeking/caregiving position to be able to interest share in a supportive, companionable way which is not dominant/submissive (p. 9).

The key to unlocking our creative potential is being able to engage in a dynamic process that is fear-free and restores our well-being to the best it can be. McCluskey (2010) believes that professions such as occupational therapy need to recognise the impact of their own fear system on themselves and their work, so that they can learn how the restorative process of attachment can reinvigorate and maintain vitality and well-being. Working with people who are seeking care for their distress brings with it intolerable emotions which can activate the professional caregiver's fear system and markedly reduce their exploratory and caregiving abilities. Similarly, Nicholls (2003, 2007), in her opinion piece, draws from the influential work of psychoanalyst and social scientist Isabel Menzies Lyth (1988). She believes that Menzies Lyth's organisational insights are still as relevant today in occupational therapy, where the profession's positive and enabling view may be harnessing defensive caregiving that wards off anxieties through manic activity. Nicholls (2003, 2007) considers that clinicians may be managing primitive anxiety around change by using comfortable and familiar patterns of activity that either deny or repress distress, exclusion and dependence. This is where clinical supervision can assist and support the therapist to recognise and regulate their own emotional defences, which can infiltrate their work (Daniel and Blair, 2002).

Assisting caregiving awareness

People seek care in a variety of ways and at times it may be difficult to know how to respond appropriately, which can leave both therapist and patient/client feeling frustrated and dissatisfied if the goal of careseeking remains unmet. To begin to assist someone with their difficulties, we first need to understand what is happening in our own bodies and how we can store up our own tensions and fears. Just as the quality of the carer/child relationship is important to the developing infant, so too is the quality of the relationship experienced in the therapeutic encounter (McCluskey, 2005). Ainsworth would liken the therapeutic relationship to the mother re-entering the room in the Strange Situation Test, as consideration needs to be given to not overwhelming the client, so that fear can be low enough to allow the person to keep exploring to maintain their well-being (Ainsworth, Blehar, Waters and Walls, 1978). Ainsworth was able to capture the fact that children play less when their mother leaves them in unfamiliar surroundings, and that a secure child will gradually return to play on her return.

From a relational perspective, Piergrossi and Gibertoni (1999) stress the importance of the internal environment for both the patient and the therapist in constructing a secure therapeutic space, where the choice of an activity can unlock expressive narratives. If fear can be lowered sufficiently, a person can move into exploratory interest sharing through choosing an activity that can absorb and that has the potential for new learning. This shifts the person into a more collaborative approach where the therapist can remain attentive and not solely centring on a careseeking/caregiving relationship (McCluskey, 2010).

When someone comes to therapy, they are often feeling anxious and alone, and the offer of assistance, from a professional caregiver, will set the attachment dynamic in motion. Therapists need to hold in mind that they can become important to the person they are treating, as a relationship has been established and issues around *attachment, separation* and *loss* will have been aroused (Bowlby, 1969/82, 1973, 1980). Previous experiences of help, however, may not have been satisfactory. These experiences will be logged within the person's internal environment as a possible outcome for this current encounter. If the fear system is aroused within the system for self-defence, the person will not be feeling safe and secure as they will be unable to use the supports on offer or may utilise them inappropriately. McCluskey notes that the therapist's caregiving system can be infiltrated by their fear system and that the therapist needs to note this in order to return to a state of exploratory caregiving towards their client (2011b).

Occupational therapists also need to focus on the doing process, by being interested and curious, available to share in the exploration of an activity, as a 'potential peer' and interested companion (Heard, Lake and McCluskey, 2009, p. 75). Una McCluskey stresses the importance of being welcomed at the start of any therapy session, to give the person a real sense of belonging. She would also emphasise the importance of therapists centring themselves before centring the other person. Being centred requires us to be as present and attentive as possible, sitting firmly in an upright, balanced position, which lifts and lengthens the spine, while paying attention to what is happening physically and emotionally within the body. In settling our own fear level, we can then tune into the altering feelings in ourselves and the other person (Heard, Lake and McCluskey, 2009; Heard, McCluskey and Lake, 2011). Just as a parent regulates an infant through the subtle movements and expressions of their body and face, a therapist, too, has to be alert to the signals going on between them as the activity unfolds (Heard, Lake and McCluskey, 2009; Heard, McCluskey and Lake, 2011). This helps to promote more effective caregiving in an environment that is as fear-free as possible, and encourages exploration without the need to interpret. For occupational therapists it is important to note that when a person feels insecure they are less inclined to explore, as their interests are no longer available to them (McCluskey, 2011b).

Conclusions

This chapter has introduced the reader to an evolving theory that has grown out of John Bowlby's ideas on attachment theory and become a new theory and practice of self, through the innovative work of Heard, Lake and McCluskey

(Heard, Lake and McCluskey, 2009; Heard, McCluskey and Lake, 2011; McCluskey, 2011a). It seems to me that it is essential for health care professionals such as occupational therapists to be aware of how their attachment and fear systems operate within both themselves and the people they aim to treat. I believe that this needs to be done by bridging the distance between people so that the greatest journey, of experiencing relationships, can be built on fear-free relating. From a psychodynamic perspective, I would consider that Brian Lake's passion for exploratory interest sharing offers occupational therapists a unique opportunity from which to explore their creative potential, through the validation received from peers and interested colleagues, and the contribution this offers in restoring well-being to a profession whose core values lie in the doing process. Whatever our age, our zest for life is generated through the exploring and sharing of interests in a supportive companionable way.

References

Ainsworth, M., Blehar, M., Waters, E., and Walls, S. (1978) *Patterns of Attachment: Assessed in the Strange Situation and at Home*. Hillsdale, NJ: Erlbaum.

Atkinson, K., and Wells, C. (2000) *Creative Therapies: A Psychodynamic Approach within Occupational Therapy*. Cheltenham: Stanley Thornes.

Balbernie, R. (2001) Circuits and circumstances: The neurobiological consequences of early relationship experiences and how they shape later behaviour. *Journal of Child Psychotherapy*, 27 (3), 237–255.

Bowlby, J. (1969/82) *Attachment and Loss (Vol. I: Attachment)*. London: Hogarth Press.

Bowlby, J. (1973) *Attachment and Loss (Vol. II: Separation: Anxiety and Anger)* London: Hogarth Press.

Bowlby, J. (1980) *Attachment and Loss (Vol. III: Loss: Sadness and Depression)* London: Hogarth Press.

Bowlby, J. (1988) *A Secure Base: Clinical Applications of Attachment Theory*. London: Hogarth Press.

Bretherton, I. (2005) In pursuit of the internal working construct and its relevance to attachment relationships. In K. E. Grossmann, K. Grossmann and E. Waters (eds), *Attachment from Infancy to Adulthood: The Major Longitudinal Studies* (pp. 13–47). New York: Guilford Press.

Daniel, M. A., and Blair, S. E. E. (2002) A psychodynamic approach to clinical supervision: 1. *British Journal of Therapy and Rehabilitation*, 9 (6), 237–240.

Fonagy, P., and Target, M. (2003) *Psychoanalytic Theories: Perspectives for Developmental Psychopathology*. London, Whurr.

Gerhardt, S. (2004) *Why Love Matters: How Affection Shapes a Baby's Brain*. London: Routledge.

Gerhardt, S. (2010) *The Selfish Society: How We All Forgot to Love One Another and Made Money Instead*. London: Simon & Schuster.

Gomez, L. (1997) *An Introduction to Object Relations*. London: Free Association.

Griffiths, S. (2008) The exploration of creative activity as a treatment medium. *Journal of Mental Health*, 17 (1), 49–63.

Grossman, K., Grossman, K., and Waters, E. (eds) (2005) *Attachment from Infancy to Adulthood: The Major Longitudinal Studies*. New York: Guilford Press.

Heard, D. (1978) From object relations to attachment theory. *British Journal of Medical Psychology*, 51, 67–76.

Heard, D. H., and Lake, B. (1986) The attachment dynamic in adult life. *British Journal of Psychiatry*, 149, 430–439.

Heard, D., and Lake, B. (1997) *The Challenge of Attachment for Caregiving.* London: Routledge.

Heard, D. H., and Lake, B. (2009) *The Challenge of Attachment for Caregiving (2nd edn)* London: Karnac.

Heard, D., Lake, B and McCluskey, U. (2009) *Attachment Therapy with Adolescents and Adults.* London: Karnac.

Heard, D., McCluskey, U., and Lake, B. (2011) *Attachment Therapy with Adolescents and Adults* (2nd edn) London: Karnac.

Hinde, R. (2005) Ethology and attachment theory. In K. Grossman, K. Grossman and E. Waters (eds), *Attachment from Infancy to Adulthood: The Major Longitudinal Studies.* New York: Guilford Press.

Holder, V. (2001) The use of creative activities within occupational therapy. *British Journal of Occupational Therapy*, 64 (2), 103–105.

Holford, A. (2011) A new way of looking at creative activities and health. *OTNews, March,* 34–35.

Holmes, J. (1993) *John Bowlby and Attachment Theory.* London: Routledge.

Holmes, J. (1994) Attachment theory: A secure theoretical base in counselling? *Psychodynamic Counselling*, 1 (1), 65–78.

Holmes, J. (1996) *Attachment, Intimacy, Autonomy: Using Attachment Theory in Adult Psychotherapy.* New Jersey/London: Jason Aronson.

Holmes, J. (2010) *Exploring in Security: Towards an Attachment-Informed Psychoanalytic Psychotherapy.* London: Routledge.

Lake, B. (1985) The concept of ego strength in psychotherapy. *British Journal of Psychiatry*, 147, 471–478.

LeDoux, J. (1998) *The Emotional Brain.* London: Weidenfeld & Nicolson.

Lemma, A. (2003) *Introduction to the Practice of Psychoanalytic Psychotherapy.* London: Wiley.

McCluskey, U. (2005) *To Be Met as a Person: The Dynamics of Attachment in Professional Encounters.* London: Karnac.

McCluskey, U. (2008) Attachment-based therapy in groups: Exploring a new paradigm with professional care-givers. *Attachment: New Directions in Psychotherapy and Relational Psychoanalysis*, 2, July, 204–215.

McCluskey, U. (2010) Understanding the self and understanding therapy: An attachment perspective. *Context*, February, 29–32.

McCluskey, U (2011a) Exploratory Goal Corrected Psychotherapy (EGCP)©. *www.unamccluskey.com* (accessed 16.04.2012).

McCluskey, U. (2011b) The therapist as a fear-free caregiver: Supporting change in the dynamic organisation of the self. *Association for University and College Counselling Journal*, May, 12–17.

Menzies Lyth, I. (1988) *Containing Anxiety in Institutions.* London: Free Association Books.

Nef (New Economics Foundation) (2008) 5 ways to well-being. http://www.neweconomics. org/publications/five-ways-well-being-evidence (accessed 10.07.12).

Nicholls, L. (2003) Occupational therapy on the couch. *Therapy Weekly*, July, 10.

Nicholls, L. E. (2007) A psychoanalytic discourse in occupational therapy. In J. Creek and A. Lawson-Porter (eds), *Contemporary Issues in Occupational Therapy: Reasoning and Reflection* (pp. 55–85). Chichester: John Wiley & Sons, Ltd.

Piergrossi, J. C., and Gibertoni, C. (1999) The importance of inner transformation in the activity process. *Occupational Therapy International*, 2, 36–47.

Reilly, M. (1974) Defining a cobweb. In M. Reilly (ed.), *Play and Exploratory Learning: Studies of Curiosity Behaviour*. Beverly Hills, CA: Sage.

Reynolds, F. (2000) Managing depression through needlecraft creative activities: A qualitative study. *The Arts in Psychotherapy*, 27 (2), 107–114.

Robertson, J. (1952) *A Two-Year-Old Goes to Hospital (film)* London: Tavistock Child Development Research Unit.

Sadlo, G. (2004) Creativity and occupation. In M. N. Molineux (ed.), *Occupation for Occupational Therapists* (pp. 90–100) Oxford: Blackwell.

Schmid, T. (ed.) (2005) *Promoting Health through Creativity: For Professionals in Health, Arts and Education*. London: Whurr.

Scottish Government (2010) *Realising Potential: An Action Plan for Allied Health Professionals in Mental Health*. Edinburgh: Scottish Government.

Shemilt, J., and Naismith, J. (2006) Psychodynamic theories II. In J. Naismith and S. Grant (eds), *College Seminar Series: Seminars in the Psychotherapies* (pp. 63–99) London: Jason Aronson.

Shilkret, R., and Shilkret, C. (2008) Attachment theory. In J. Berzoff, L. M. Flanagan and P. Hertz (eds), *Inside Out and Outside In: Psychodynamic Clinical Theory and Psychopathology in Contemporary Multicultural Contexts* (pp. 189–203). New Jersey/London: Jason Aronson.

Stern, D. (1985) *The Interpersonal World of the Infant*. New York: Basic Books.

Thomson, M., and Blair, S. E. E. (1998) Creative arts in occupational therapy: Ancient history or contemporary practice? *Occupational Therapy International*, 5 (1), 49–65.

Timmons, A., and MacDonald, E. (2008) Alchemy and magic: The experience of using clay for people with chronic illness and disability. *British Journal of Occupational Therapy*, 71 (3), 86–94.

Winnicott, D. W. (1971) *Playing and Reality*. London: Tavistock.

6 Re-awakening Psychoanalytic Thinking in Occupational Therapy: From Gail Fidler to Here

Julie Cunningham Piergrossi

Introduction

I met Gail Fidler in person in a 3-week summer course at Boston University in 1971. I still have very clear memories of her presence, made up of elegance, energy and wonderful relational capacities. She wanted us to think about 'doing' in all of its complex dimensions, starting out with what it meant to each of us. Required reading was the book by the psychoanalyst Harold Searles, *The Nonhuman Environment in Schizophrenia and Normal Development* (1960) and the course was a combination of activity participation, discussion and writing. Gail was very generous in talking about her own experiences and created a warm and intellectually stimulating atmosphere in those 3 weeks of full immersion, which left a lasting impression on my way of understanding the possibilities of occupational therapy. My life was in Italy, so I never saw her again, but we had several communications, both written and by phone, in the years that followed and I read all of her articles and books. Her passion for the psychodynamic aspects of our profession was part of what encouraged me to undertake my own psychoanalytic training and has been fundamental for my clinical work as well as in teaching.

This chapter examines the thoughts of Gail Fidler and others who have pursued psychoanalytic theory in their work as occupational therapists. It highlights the growth and change in psychoanalytic thinking since the seminal Fidler book written with her husband in 1963, and proposes continued research in an area which should not be forgotten and might be able to re-awaken interest in giving more space to relational and emotional issues in therapy.

Psychoanalytic Thinking in Occupational Therapy: Symbolic, Relational and Transformative, First Edition.
Lindsey Nicholls, Julie Cunningham Piergrossi, Carolina de Sena Gibertoni and Margaret A. Daniel.
© 2013 John Wiley & Sons, Ltd. Published 2013 by John Wiley & Sons, Ltd.

The lasting concepts introduced by Fidler: occupation and relationship

What exactly were the core concepts of Fidler's work in the early years? She and her husband, a psychoanalyst, wrote two books together (1954, 1963). The second (*Occupational Therapy: A Communication Process in Psychiatry*) remained the sole text for occupational therapists working in mental health, for many years. They wrote about 'doing' as part of the communication process between therapist and patient, and carefully examined the specific characteristics of the various activities, which included the symbolic and unconscious significance of materials, objects and products in both individual and group approaches. Theirs was an occupational approach in the sense that it always included activities in a treatment scenario which was by definition relational because of its psychodynamic theory base. Occupation and relationship (communication, as they called it) are the lasting concepts which are still present and useful in the profession today.

Over the years, Gail Fidler's writing began to take on the larger issues of the profession, especially teaching and supervision. It is interesting to note, however, that although she seemed gradually to draw away from a strictly psychodynamic approach, I would dare to say that her early training influenced her way of envisaging teaching and learning throughout her life.

In her Eleanor Clark Slagle lecture of 1966 (the prestigious annual award of the American Occupational Therapy Association) entitled 'Learning as a growth process: A conceptual framework for professional education,' she seemed already to be taking a new path, leaving behind the purely clinical work of her recently published book. At the same time, she spoke about teaching and learning using activities, and brought in the importance of feelings and self-awareness, thus keeping alive the core concepts of occupation and relationship.

> As the activity is pursued, the students are encouraged to identify feelings which occur, explore the specific characteristics of both the action and objects which seem to elicit such feelings and discern how feelings are manifested in behaviour and in the content of productions. Involvement such as this teaches in a personally significant way the very basic concepts of occupational therapy, initiates a receptivity to self-awareness, sharpens sensitivity and understanding and thus creates the basis for an ultimately more accurate and sensitive appreciation of patient response.
>
> (Fidler, 1966, p. 149)

In this quote Fidler is describing what she calls the activity laboratory, and she presented it again (Fidler and Velde, 1999) in the book, *Activities: Reality and Symbol*. She introduces the chapter by quoting Eric Erikson when he says, 'Every human expression means more than it seems' (p. 27) and goes on to explain how the laboratory can be used to introduce groups of any kind to the richness of activities and how their characteristics elicit particular and subjective thoughts, feelings and behaviours. She wrote about 'doing' in everyday life, and in 1978 she and her husband wrote a much quoted article entitled, 'Doing and becoming: Purposeful action and self-actualization', in which they examined occupational performance as 'the ability, throughout the life cycle, to care for and maintain the self in a more independent manner, satisfy one's personal needs for intrinsic gratification, and contribute to the needs and welfare of others' (Fidler and Fidler, 1978, p. 89).

At this point they were interested in 'becoming' as a form of adaptation to the problems of everyday life and saw 'doing' as the way adaptation became possible. In her book written with Beth Velde, *Activities: Reality and Symbol* (1999), Gail continued her quest for understanding the meaning of doing and concentrated on the symbolic significance of activity. She was interested in how objects, materials and the activities themselves could express meaning linked to one's inner world and could communicate significance without using words: 'A symbol is not a proxy for its object, condition, or event. It is a "carrier" of a concept; it conveys a meaning; it communicates a thought, an abstract idea. Symbols always contain an affective element' (Fidler and Velde, 1999, p. 3).

Susan Fine (1999), in the same book, wrote: 'Acknowledging the unconscious inner life in the context of today's dynamic biopsychosocial dialectic does not commit one to the couch. It simply, and profoundly, opens the door to a *fuller understanding of how human activities at one level influence processes at another*' (p. 13).

Together with Beth Velde, Gail developed a model called 'Lifestyle performance', which the authors describe as a way of engaging the power of occupation defined as a congruence between the characteristics of an individual and the characteristics of an activity (Velde and Fidler, 2002). It is the importance given to the individual and his or her choices (lifestyle) which seem to me to bring us back to some basic psychodynamic concepts, such as personal choice, responsibility and search for the self.

In a short article written with Nedra Gillette shortly before her death, Gail wrote about her passion for understanding activity's influence on human behaviour, for teaching and for questioning in a continual give and take with learners of any age and states: 'I believe that there *are* no right answers. I therefore believe as well that each and every guiding assumption must be continually re-examined and challenged anew' (Fidler and Gillette, 2005, p. 633).

When Gail passed away in 2005, Wendy Wood (2005) remembered her as a 'questioner', someone who acted as an agent of change, upending the status quo, albeit constructively. Gillette (2005) remembered her as a mentor: 'Whoever you were, whatever you wanted to do, Gail was there to challenge you to think bigger, to think in terms of societal need, not just with regard to the issue of the moment. As our mentor, no "learner" was ever finished in Gail's mind; she was never content to leave your ideas alone' (p. 609).

In the same commemorative article, Gillette remembered Gail's interest in the unconscious and how she explored symbols. She described Gail's appreciation for the unconscious as a protective force for the client, who was struggling with losses sustained through physical injury and the life-changing adjustments required by chronic illness and disability. In these situations, fantasies, dreams and creative activities were recognised as a strong part of a sense of self, as important as reality-oriented activities.

When I began writing about Gail Fidler and her influence on psychoanalytic thinking in the profession, I was somewhat perplexed by what I viewed as her abandonment of psychodynamic practice. The kind of clinical approach she described with her husband in 1963 seemed to have disappeared from her writing. But after a close study of her way of thinking in later writing, I have changed my opinion, because I firmly believe that questioning, not-knowing, giving space to unconscious and symbolic understanding, all of which were part of her way of being (as described by Wood and Gillette above), are fundamental concepts for psychoanalytic thinking in occupational therapy. In addition, Gail Fidler never abandoned doing, occupation and activity, as part of every therapeutic relationship.

The unconscious: fear and fascination

Why are some of us so interested in unconscious phenomena, in the intricacies of emotional ambivalence, in understanding suffering, while others prefer observing behaviour, managing emotion and overcoming suffering? There is, of course, no real answer to the question, but those of us who are part of the interested group tend to see the others as perhaps fearful to look beyond the surface (the conscious explanation) of what human nature is all about. Those who prefer the observable, more concrete aspects of helping others tend to see us interested ones as unrealistic and somewhat antiquated, without clear goals or results. The unconscious is that part of the human spirit which is the object of interest to the authors of this book, that important part of the story we don't know. As Nicholls (2007) wrote about occupational therapy:

> Perhaps the most profound loss in our current discourse has been an appreciation of the unconscious and the effect that it can have on the actions and choices of individuals and within society. In the current climate of evidence-based practice and measurable outcomes that are reliant on positivist views of science and therapy, there has been a loss of wonder and delight in (appreciation of) the imaginative potential of the unconscious with its capacity to repair, reconcile and recover. The unconscious carries within it not only instinctual drives, and their concomitant anxiety, but also a capacity for connection, knowledge, wisdom and creativity.   (p. 56)

We have already seen how important the unconscious is in Gail Fidler's thinking. She states, 'Effective use of the one-to-one or group relationships and activities in treatment can occur only to the extent that one has an understanding of the impact of the unconscious' (Fidler and Fidler, 1963, p. 118). The work of the Fidlers came at a time when psychoanalytic influence on occupational therapy in mental health settings was strong. In the 1960s, when I was studying occupational therapy, about half of the theoretical and practical part of our training was dedicated to mental health concerns. Psychiatrists who taught the medical courses and who headed the hospitals where we did field work were psychoanalytically trained. People with mental illnesses were cared for in large, closed mental hospitals. Effective anti-psychotic drugs, which would have a significant impact on length of stay and symptoms, were still in the future. Our mental health training concentrated on activity participation and understanding the meaning of the activities as part of the therapeutic relationship.

Bruce and Borg (2002) state that, in occupational therapy, the psychoanalytic or psychodynamic approach in mental health was particularly strong from the 1950s through to the beginning of the 1970s. These authors give a very comprehensive outline of the psychodynamic frame of reference during those years and underline the importance given to the inner world of the patient.

> *An enduring contribution of a psychodynamic framework has been that it alerts occupational therapists to attend to the emotional or affective part of the person. It reminds us as occupational therapists that sometimes what our client thinks or knows may be quite different from what he or she feels, and that feelings exert a powerful influence on people's choices, motivation and continued engagement in occupation.*
>
> (Bruce and Borg, 2002, p. 71)

Another example of respect for the unconscious in our profession was in the extensive use of projective techniques for evaluation purposes, using clay, painting and collage among other materials in working with mental health clients (Hemphill, 1982). Eklund (2000) describes and proposes the use of a projective test called PORT, the Percept-genetic Object Relation Test, for assessing patients' internal object relations.

The role of the unconscious is very present in an interesting article on the value of client resistance in occupational therapy (Davis, 2007), which presents the psycho-dynamic hypothesis that resistance does not obstruct therapy but is rather the stuff of therapy, and suggests the need for research to explore occupational therapists' subjective judgements concerning client resistance.

Psychoanalytically trained occupational therapists

There are perhaps three ways in which psychoanalytically trained occupational therapists tend to contribute to our profession: supervision and teaching (Daniel and Blair, 2002; Mackenzie and Beecraft, 2004); analysis of the culture of the profession itself; and emphasis on re-engaging with psychoanalytic knowledge and applying psychoanalytic concepts to occupational therapy practice and research (Nicholls, 2007; Finlay, 1998) and clinical practice (Cunningham Piergrossi, 2010; Gibertoni, 2006; Cunningham Piergrossi and Gibertoni, 1995; Eklund, 2000; Ainscough, 1998). Probably all of these people are active in two if not in all three of these ways of being psychoanalytic occupational therapists, but they tend to concentrate their writing and research in one of the three areas.

In the course of the last 45 years, psychodynamic occupational therapy has stayed alive thanks to those of us who have remained committed to its central tenets for one reason or another, perhaps more so in Europe than in the United States. In Italy, where psychoanalysis was thriving during the 1970s and 1980s, a small group of occupational therapists was carrying on with clinical work based on psychoanalytic theory and initiated by Gail Fidler's teaching. They were untouched by the health care forces changing the profession in the USA and UK. The possibility of sharing ideas with others about 'doing' as part of the therapeutic relationship led to an ever more enlarged field and brought creative ways of working and thinking (Cunningham Piergrossi and Gibertoni, 1995, 2005). I am particularly thankful to Carolina Gibertoni and all she taught me about the power of emotion and the theories of the English psychoanalysts encountered in her own training at the Tavistock Clinic in London. In 2006 Carolina published a book called *Cibo per pensare: La cucina terapeutica con bambini e adolescenti* (Food for Thought: Therapeutic Cooking with Children and Adolescents), which beautifully illustrates how psychoanalytic thinking can help human beings in general and sick children in particular to get on with their lives and their significant occupations.

A Swedish occupational therapist, Mona Eklund, has been writing for many years about object relations theory applied to our profession (1996, 1998, 2000) and proposes an object relations model for occupational therapy. Eklund (2000) uses the theories of Sullivan and Winnicott together with the American relationalists Greenberg and Mitchell as a base for building the model, and underlines the importance of relationships as part of occupations. She demonstrates how the relational model within object relations theory seems to have an inherent broad link to occupational therapy. 'It stems from psychodynamic psychology and social psychology and assumes an innate need to relate to others as present in all humans. How this need is met determines the individual's development and psychosocial behaviour' (2000, p. 15). Eklund distinguishes between short-term and long-term therapy and both explicit and implicit methods for occupational therapy. She emphasises the necessity for research which goes beyond the empirical evidence of randomised controlled trials and quantitative measures.

The field of creative therapies in the United Kingdom is covered by Kim Atkinson and Catherine Wells in their book entitled *Creative Therapies: A Psychodynamic Approach within Occupational Therapy* (2000). The authors describe in precise detail their work with groups of adults using creative activities which include painting, body movement, clay and sculpture, sound and rhythm, and text and verse. 'In creative therapy the product is implicit, achieved through a process of self-discovery, self-exploration, self-determination and self-help' (p. 295). The method they describe in the book encourages therapists to prepare a therapy session proposing specific activities, but giving maximum space to individual expression. It was very interesting to me that with one of their groups they propose making a pizza in one of the group sessions to overcome a difficult conflictual moment. They explain that this flexibility in using a variety of activities as the situation demands is the principal difference between occupational therapy and other forms of creative therapy.

Changes in psychoanalysis itself

Psychoanalysis has always been practised in different forms according to the school, country and time in which the analyst is trained. Occupational therapists, like everyone else, have been influenced by the colleagues with whom we work, our own psychoanalytic training, and the country in which we live. What is important for us as a profession is to use the ideas of psychoanalysis which are particularly applicable and important for understanding human participation in meaningful occupation.

I have sometimes found the references in occupational therapy literature to the use of psychoanalysis in our profession as having a mechanistic approach, using a medical model and based on some of the earliest Freudian treatment and theoretical concepts (e.g. Sharrott, 1986; Barris, Keilhofner and Watts, 1983). I was struck by the narrow and extremely critical way they used to describe something that for me had opened unknown worlds of wonder about the nature of what it is to be human. Psychoanalytic thinking offers questions and not answers about existential quandaries that have been fascinating humankind for a long time. What I have realised in my reading is that there are many misconceptions about psychoanalysis and that these are largely due to a lack of knowledge about what has been happening in this discipline over the last 50 years. In order to understand how we have arrived at this point in the long voyage from Fidler to here, we must also look at what has been happening in psychoanalysis in general. It is not in the scope of this chapter to review the vast psychoanalytic literature available on the subject, but I would like to try to summarise briefly the observations that I find very pertinent for occupational therapy based on my own experience in Italy, on theory presented in other chapters of this book and on theories of other contemporary analysts.

First of all, there has been a gradual shift from concentrating on alleviating the specific pathology or symptoms of the patient to concentrating on the relationship between patient and analyst.

Secondly, the patient's suffering is respected and contained by the analyst. His or her resources are recognised, but first of all their mental pain is accepted, contained and shared.

Another important change has been the confluence of neurobiological studies and psychoanalytical research, meaning that there is no longer a rigid dichotomy between biological and psychological explanations for mental phenomena. Seigel (1999) writes about recent findings of neural science, 'Interactions with the environment, especially relationships with other people, directly shape the development of the brain's structure and function. There is no need to choose between brain or mind, biology or experience, nature or nurture. These divisions are unhelpful and inhibit clear thinking about an important and complex subject: the developing human mind' (p. x).

A fourth point has to do with the use of self and, more precisely, the difficult subject of self-revelation on the part of the analyst, which is being taken into consideration in new ways by many psychoanalysts. Lewis Aron (1996) writes, 'Self-revelation is not an option: it is an inevitability' (p. 84). He describes the position of the analyst in the use of self: 'A dynamic tension needs to be preserved between responsiveness and participation, on one hand, and nonintrusiveness and space on the other, intermediate between the analyst's presence and absence' (p. 87).

Lastly, one of the goals of psychoanalysis is to help the patient to be able to take responsibility for his or her life. I am not talking about enabling empowerment here, but about a therapist free from judgement who is promoting a firm sense of self in the patient, who becomes more able to make his or her own choices.

An enlarged field: from the Fidler approach to the development of the MOVI

In preparing this chapter and reading and rereading the pertinent literature, I am struck by a seeming contradiction in my feelings. I can clearly see the similarities between the early teaching of Gail Fidler and the application of her model to the work I am still doing today. In fact, I think to myself that if someone were to look into the window of my therapy room, they would see the same kind of work I was doing 45 years ago. What they would not see is the way I think about what I do and they would not hear the things I say to my patients. A recent simple example can better explain what I mean.

> ### Paolo learning to use a saw: a harmony of force and skill
>
> Ten-year-old Paolo was building a box with wood and having difficulty finding the right use of force both for sawing and for drilling holes with the hand drill. I talked to him about how with wood it is necessary to find the right balance between the force of strength and the lightness of touch with the tools. Paolo is a boy who comes to me for problems in controlling his rage, which causes him enormous problems both at home and at school; and he accuses me of not controlling his anger for him. The work with the wood gave me the chance to ask myself if, in anger, there is not something similar that happens – not only a question of making it disappear, but with lightness of touch being able to modify its force somehow and use it in a constructive way. And in the meantime Paolo really learned during that session to saw the wood in a harmonious way without exhausting himself, bending the blade or badly breaking the wood. Something happened between him, me and the woodworking that helped me to be nearer to his anger in a way that he could begin to feel and to use.

As I reread the Fidler book, the differences between it and my way of thinking and working today became clear to me and seemed enormously significant. They all have to do with the relationship between therapist, patient and 'doing' in the here and now of each therapy session. I have identified three aspects of the MOVI (described in detail in Chapter 7) and compared them with the approach described by the Fidlers in their 1963 book, as a way of demonstrating how time and hard work have enlarged the field of psychoanalytic occupational therapy, enabling it to grow and to change.

The three areas of development in theory and clinical practice are: the transformation process during the participation in activities; choice as a fixed part of the structure of the setting; and the importance of the therapist's feelings in the therapeutic process.

The examples given here illustrate what I consider an extension of Gail Fidler's work and follow a trend that has affected the whole field of psychoanalysis. Fidler started us thinking about psychoanalysis in occupational therapy, and then experience and training led us to a whole new way of understanding the 'doing' as part of the relationship between occupational therapist and patient. I have included the thoughts of authors who have helped me to reflect further on the three concepts. The influences of the theories of Freud, Bion, Klein and Winnicott are not included here since complete chapters in this book (see Chapters 3 and 4) are dedicated to their contribution to the MOVI (Chapter 7).

The transformation process: standing in the spaces with Anna

The Fidlers (1963) saw activities as facilitating the communication process between therapist and patient:

> *In occupational therapy the psychodynamics of activities are considered as catalytic agents giving impetus to the development of relationships and intrapsychic experiences, which are used by the therapist and patient collaboratively to alter and eliminate pathology. By process we refer to the stimuli of the real and symbolic meaning of an object or activity, the intrapsychic responses of the patient to such stimuli, the pervading influence that such feeling, thinking, and acting has on interpersonal relationships, and the collaborative efforts and communication between patient and therapist.*
>
> (p. 118)

I was glad to see the similarities between the words of the Fidlers and the MOVI, a model that views activities as initiating a transformation process which begins with the transformation of materials, but which includes a parallel process leading to an inner transformation. The action on the materials being used begins to ferry emotions and memories which are not immediately evident and available to the conscious mind. Perhaps we can say that this aspect has now become central to the whole process of activity participation and hence to occupational therapy's unique contribution to alleviating human emotional suffering. In the MOVI, the therapist's attention goes first to the activity choice, followed by participation, comprehension and communication. An example of this process can be found in the story of Anna, a 14-year-old girl who came to occupational therapy after she had prematurely ended three previous individual psychotherapy experiences. She was a very bright girl, read a lot, had normal relationships with her peers but had refused to go to school for the past 3 years. She lived with her father, having lost her mother, who committed suicide when Anna was 4 years old.

Anna's wooden block

Anna chooses wood carving, a new activity for her, and decides to make a small box. Technically this is a difficult task: she must gouge with force and precision, and accept the slowness of a long project. Sliver after sliver, she cuts out the inner space of the small container, and towards the end of the session she begins to talk about being hospitalised after the death of her mother for a spinal tap because they thought she had a serious illness. She tells about how she had become completely blocked, as hard as a piece of wood; that she moved rigidly as if her body were all one piece. She begins to talk about the death of her mother and the shocking scene she remembers having seen. We can hypothesise that the aggressive cutting with the tool in the wood reminded her of the fear of the spinal tap, which for a young child was certainly painful and invasive. It is interesting that she describes herself as 'blocked and rigid like a piece of wood'. She uses this expression after 30 minutes of concentrated carving in the hard material of wood. We can imagine that, as she transformed the rough material into a small box, gouge after gouge, there was a parallel movement inside herself which transformed an emotional block into a space for being able to remember, to think and to tell.

Anna accepted the occupational therapy approach whereas she had refused psychotherapy, probably because occupational therapy provided her with a distance from the therapist and 'doing' something may have offered an alternative to talking. But 'doing' also offered a symbolic connection to her inner world because it was in the transformation of the wood that an inner transformation was put in motion as well, kindling memories and emotions that she had never talked about with anyone.

I was reminded of Philip Bromberg's work on trauma and dissociation (1998). Bromberg, an American psychoanalyst, wrote a book entitled *Standing in the Spaces*. He considers dissociation a natural phenomenon in human living and only pathological when we are unable to be in some conscious contact with our various self states. Anna had completely dissociated her suffering 'rigid like a piece of wood' self, saying that lots of people had mothers who died young. She began to 'see' this self as she carved the wood for her little box and together with a therapist who was ready to receive her very precious and traumatic memories. The woodworking and the relationship with the therapist had helped her to stand in the spaces of her different self states. The first sentence of Bromberg's book begins like this: 'I've always been wary of words . . .' (p. 1). He begins this way to explain his own 'ability to disappear inside himself, as if in another world' (p. 1), and he continues to explain what he sees as the 'heart of personality growth – the paradox of being known but still remaining private, of being in the world but still separate from it' (p. 1). This describes Anna very well, but the unconscious part of her being separate from the world was interfering with one of the most important occupations for a 14-year-old, that of attending school as part of a peer group.

Fidler's early work (Fidler and Fidler, 1963) also speaks to materials and activities reaching unconscious forces, and she analysed carefully what patients expressed through their actions on materials. What has been added now is the importance of uniting the action with the materials to what is happening at the same time with the therapist, not as a sequential process but in a simultaneous mode.

Choice as a fixed part of the structure of the setting: Valeria

The patient's choice of activities in the occupational therapy sessions, as described in the Fidlers' book, was always taken into consideration and so had a similar meaning to how it is seen in the MOVI, but it was not a fixed part of the setting itself. For the Fidlers, choice as an indication of personal difference and subjectivity was highly respected; however, they did not write about accepting and using difficult or negative choices as part of the therapeutic process. In the MOVI, the concept of choice becomes a dynamic part of the setting itself, because it is the therapist who offers the patient the chance to choose from the many materials and activities in the room. The therapist is less concerned about what the specific choice might be and more concentrated on what happens when there is a therapist who offers a choice, and what this means in the relationship and within the boundary of place and time.

Valeria's unfinished objects

Twelve-year-old Valeria, part of a small group, was creative and artistically talented but never finished the beautiful objects she began, leaving them in the therapy room half completed. Clay sculptures, paintings, leather purses and wooden ships would take on harmonious shapes and show promise of delightful results, only to be abandoned shortly thereafter by their creator. My role was difficult because I realised I had to accept Valeria's choice not to finish her products and put aside my strong desire to encourage her to do so. She was surrounded in her life by adults who were constantly insisting that she live up to her true capabilities, reprimanding her for her messiness and her inconclusiveness. Her teachers and family wanted her to be more responsible, but Valeria, who had lost both parents and was presently living with her aunt, was in a much younger emotional stage of development. Her confusion and uncertainty were reflected in her partial objects, and I realised I had to accept the way she thought of herself, with a sense of identity only half-formed, like the objects she produced. It was a clear way of letting her know that in our work together she could be herself. If I had insisted on the necessity of completing her products, it would have been like saying, 'I don't like you the way you are now; I want you to be different.' Valeria was free to choose the incompleteness of her products and her sense of responsibility would arrive when she was surer of her own completeness.

Choice in the Fidlers' way of viewing activities in therapy could be either positive or negative. As pointed out by Nicholls (2007):

> They [the Fidlers] suggested that we need to analyse the patient's actions and choices in order to encourage different activities that can promote growth and maturity ... What the authors have ignored is that the choice of occupation is a symbolic representation of inner and outward processes and that changing the overt manifestation of this struggle will not change the impulse (drive) for the activity.

(p. 62)

When choice is part of the structure of the setting, as in the MOVI, all choices must be honoured, whatever they may be, as long as they don't go against the rules of safety for all persons involved. This means that the therapist is always ready to question choices, to talk about them, to understand their meaning together with the patient, but always in a non-judgemental way. When Valeria chose for a long time to not finish her products, I was able to communicate my acceptance of a part of her that was constantly criticised by others, and she was more able to really look at herself instead of simply acting out her repetitive opposition to adults, a category of human beings she was not yet ready to trust.

Janis Davis (2007), an occupational therapist writing about the value of resistance, seemed to illuminate another way of understanding Valeria's unfinished products:

> *A willingness to tolerate uncomfortable feelings and go forward without a therapeutic agenda allows therapists to go where their clients wish to go. Wishing is the first step on the road to action. Therapists who explore their own feelings, have the courage to look at their level of professional competence, and the search for the value in resistance will empower clients to work on their own behalf. It is this newfound power that may turn a wish into a reality.*
>
> (p. 52)

The importance of the therapist's feelings: the therapy process with Lucia

I found no references in the Fidler book to the therapist using her own feelings to better understand her patient. It must be remembered that the understanding and use of countertransference has developed over the last 30 years in psychoanalysis. In the MOVI, the feelings of the therapist are a fundamental part of the therapy itself because they can indicate the ways in which the 'doing' links the inner world of the therapist with the inner world of the patient. What I am describing here is not countertransference as such, but rather an inner movement of emotions on the part of both of the participants in the relationship.

Lucia: Learning to be present

The first time I heard Lucia's story I felt a strong sense of anguish (probably partially due to the fact of having a daughter of about the same age), and it was this very anguish which enabled me to finally feel close and to be able to help her, but only after a long process that involved both of us. This lovely 27-year-old woman had suffered a severe brain trauma 2 years earlier which erased all of her memory from before the accident. When she was hit by a car while riding her bicycle, Lucia had just finished her fifth year of medical school. A month of coma left her with partial paralysis on her right side and without language. She had started all over and in fact many times during her therapy she would repeat, 'I died and came back to life another person.' Now after physical therapy, speech therapy and various medical and psychological interventions, she still has had no return of memory from before the accident, has some difficulty with recent memory and has some cognitive impairment. She has learned to write and paint with her left hand and is independent in her movements and daily activities. She takes watercolour painting and ceramic classes, but has lost all of her friends from before the accident and even sees her twin sister very rarely. She lives with her parents, who help her, encourage her and include her in their activities, but who still seem without resources for coping with the loss of the 'Lucia from before'.

My goals with Lucia from the beginning had to do with her request of 'finding herself'. I hoped that through participation in activities chosen by her I would be able to help her concentrate on and accept the present Lucia. I was very aware of the fact that I only knew the 'now' Lucia, and this gave me a kind of advantage over the other people in her life, who communicated a quiet desperation whenever I spoke with them because of the differences in her, particularly in cognitive abilities, after the accident.

She liked coming to occupational therapy, but my containment function was difficult because it was very hard for her to take in what came from others. She talked and she listened, but she tended to do and say things that she knew the other person wanted to hear, having little capacity for reflection and elaboration of her thoughts. She had a personal story book where she would write poetry, paint and draw, creating memories that were shared with me as an important part of our relationship.

What I want to underline here is the importance for me of coming to terms with my own emotions regarding Lucia and the things she chose to do and how she did them, in order to be able to help her. Lucia had a sweet and positive personality, but her slowness and her tendency to concentrate all of her energy on the moment of the accident and on her 'death' made the therapy sessions terribly repetitive and I found myself sluggish, sleepy and bored. It seemed like I was doing absolutely nothing for her. I brought my difficulties to supervision with psychoanalyst colleagues who helped me to realise how much the sense of slowness and emptiness I was experiencing was reflecting what was happening in Lucia and was weighing on the therapy sessions. When at a certain point several members of the group suggested terminating the therapy, I felt a deep and profound sadness, an identification with my patient that helped me to realise what was behind the emptiness that had blocked us both. After this insight into my own feelings of sadness, I was able to continue her therapy with a much freer capacity for thought, which is probably when I was finally able to help Lucia to start moving towards the future.

In present psychoanalytic literature, the therapist's emotions, memories and thoughts are considered a valuable part of the relationship (Aron, 1996; Bromberg,

2006). For occupational therapists who work with a psychoanalytic orientation, this very complex phenomenon must be acknowledged and enlarged upon to include the 'doing' and the materials that are part of our setting.

Gail Fidler helped us to see doing as a valuable asset in communicating with our patients. Occupational therapy today, based on doing as a dynamic process that touches the inner worlds of all of the participants, has added another dimension to therapy, more complex, multifaceted and requiring psychoanalytic training and supervision to be able to fully appreciate and apply its potential. What has come about is a fascinating way of carrying out therapy, raising more questions than giving answers – exactly what Gail Fidler hoped would happen as a result of her teaching.

Conclusions

I have been thinking recently about Gail Fidler and what she would think about the book we have written and her part in it. I remember her words in one of our last conversations when she told me she had changed her ideas, as I was telling her about our psychoanalytically based work in Italy. I think now she would be pleased to know that a seed she had planted had grown into something she had not foreseen. And isn't that the most exciting thing that can happen for a teacher?

References

Ainscough, K. (1998) The therapeutic value of activity in child psychiatry. *British Journal of Occupational Therapy*, 61 (5), 223–226.

Aron, L. (1996) *A Meeting of Minds: Mutuality in Psychoanalysis*. Hillsdale, NJ: The Analytic Press.

Atkinson, K., and Wells, C. (2000) *Creative Therapies: A Psychodynamic Approach within Occupational Therapy*. Cheltenham: Stanley Thornes.

Barris, R., Keilhofner, G., and Watts, J. (1983) *Psychosocial Occupational Therapy: Practice in a Pluralistic Arena*. Laurel: Ramsco.

Bromberg, P. (1998) *Standing in the Spaces*. Hillsdale, NJ: The Analytic Press.

Bromberg, P. (2006) *Awakening the Dreamer*. Hillsdale, NJ: The Analytic Press.

Bruce, M., and Borg, B. (2002) *Frames of Reference in Psychosocial Occupational Therapy*. Thorofare, NJ: Slack.

Cunningham Piergrossi, J. (2010) Expressing cultural identity through choice, memory and emotion. *South African Journal of Occupational Therapy*, supplement, August.

Cunningham Piergrossi, J., and Gibertoni, C. de Sena (1995) The importance of inner transformation in the activity process. *Occupational Therapy International*, 2 (1), 36–47.

Cunningham Piergrossi, J., and Gibertoni, C. de Sena (2005) The interactive process and mental functions in occupational therapy. *WFOT Bulletin*, 52, 25–28.

Daniel, M., and Blair, S. (2002) A psychodynamic approach to clinical supervision: 1. *British Journal of Therapy and Rehabilitation*, 9 (6), 237–240.

Davis, J. (2007) Finding value in client resistance. *Occupational Therapy in Mental Health*, 23 (1), 39–54.

Eklund, M. (1996) Patient experiences and outcome of treatment in psychiatric occupational therapy – three cases. *Occupational Therapy International*, 3, 138–165.

Eklund, M. (1998) Outcome of occupational therapy treatment in a psychiatric day care unit for long-term mentally ill patients. *Occupational Therapy in Mental Health*, 14, 21–45.

Eklund, M. (2000) Applying object relations theory to psychosocial occupational therapy: Empirical and theoretical considerations. *Occupational Therapy in Mental Health*, 15 (1), 1–26.

Fidler, G. (1966) Learning as a growth process: A conceptual framework for professional education. *American Journal of Occupational Therapy*, 20 (1), 1–8.

Fidler, G., and Fidler, J. (1954) *Introduction to Psychiatric Occupational Therapy*. New York: Macmillan.

Fidler, G., and Fidler, J. (1963) *Occupational Therapy: A Communication Process in Psychiatry*. New York: Macmillan.

Fidler, G., and Fidler. J. (1978) Doing and becoming: Purposeful action and self-actualization. *American Journal of Occupational Therapy*, 32 (5), 305–310.

Fidler, G., and Gillette, N. (2005) Passion and perseverance. *American Journal of Occupational Therapy*, 59 (6), 632–633.

Fidler, G., and Velde, B. (1999) *Activities: Reality and Symbol*. Thorofare, NJ: Slack.

Fine, S. (1999) Symbolization: Making meaning for self and society. In G. Fidler and B. Velde (eds), *Activities: Reality and Symbol* (pp. 11–26) Thorofare, NJ: Slack.

Finlay, L. (1998) Reflexivity: An essential component for all research? *British Journal of Occupational Therapy*, 61 (10), 453–456.

Gibertoni, C. (2006) *Cibo per pensare: La cucina terapeutica con bambini e adolescenti*. Rome: Borla.

Gillette, N. (2005) A tribute to Gail S. Fidler, our esteemed mentor. *American Journal of Occupational Therapy*, 59 (6), 609–610.

Hemphill, B. (1982) *The Evaluative Process in Psychiatric Occupational Therapy*. Thorofare, NJ: Slack.

Mackenzie, A., and Beecraft, S. (2004) The use of psychodynamic observation as a tool for learning and reflective practice when working with older adults. *British Journal of Occupational Therapy*, 67 (12), 533–539.

Nicholls, L. (2007) A psychoanalytic discourse in occupational therapy. In *Contemporary Issues in Occupational Therapy* (pp. 55–86) Chichester: John Wiley & Sons, Ltd.

Searles, H. (1960) *The Nonhuman Environment in Normal Development and in Schizophrenia*. New York: International Universities Press.

Seigel, D. (1999) *The Developing Mind*. New York: Guildford Press.

Sharrott, G. (1986) An analysis of occupational therapy theoretical approaches for mental health: Are the profession's major treatment approaches truly occupational therapy? *Occupational Therapy in Mental Health*, 5 (4), 1–16.

Velde, B., and Fidler, G. (2002) *Lifestyle Performance: A Model for Engaging the Power of Occupation*. Thorofare, NJ: Slack.

Wood, W. (2005) A firm persuasion in our work – Editor's note – Question or settle? *American Journal of Occupational Therapy*, 59 (6), 631.

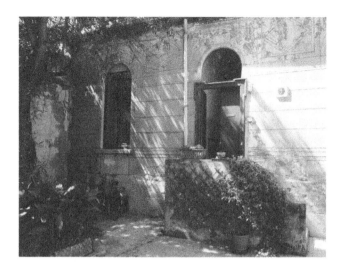

The Vivaio house, Milan. Photograph taken by J. Cunningham.

Section 2

Psychoanalytic Occupational Therapy: A Relational Practice Model and Illuminating Theory in Clinical Practice

This section introduces the reader to the MOVI (Chapter 7), a relational practice model in occupational therapy. It is currently the only occupational therapy model that incorporates an understanding of the unconscious in what is done and said (or not said) within the therapeutic encounter between the client, the occupational therapist and the activity. This chapter is pivotal within the book, and is informed by psychoanalytic theory and informs occupational therapy practice and training.

Chapters 8 and 9 cover areas of specialist interest: understanding the effects on the clients and therapists when working in the area of child abuse; and working with 'difference' in organisational contexts. Both the authors have used psychoanalytic theory to discuss these two areas in some depth and relate this thinking to clinical examples.

Psychoanalytic Thinking in Occupational Therapy: Symbolic, Relational and Transformative, First Edition.
Lindsey Nicholls, Julie Cunningham Piergrossi, Carolina de Sena Gibertoni and Margaret A. Daniel.
© 2013 John Wiley & Sons, Ltd. Published 2013 by John Wiley & Sons, Ltd.

7 MOVI: A Relational Model in Occupational Therapy

Julie Cunningham Piergrossi and Carolina de Sena Gibertoni

Introduction: how MOVI was developed

This chapter will describe the Vivaio model (MOVI), an occupational therapy relational model of practice with a psychoanalytic theory base. MOVI is currently the only occupational therapy practice model that incorporates an understanding of the unconscious in what is done and said (or not said) within the therapeutic encounter between the client, the occupational therapist and the activity. It brings back into view the early work of Fidler and Fidler (1963) and has been built on the clinical observations and reflections of this chapter's authors, Cunningham Piergrossi and Gibertoni.

MOVI was born and grew in three rooms in an old and romantic courtyard in the middle of the city of Milan, Italy, surrounded by oleander trees and peeling walls. The name of the centre was 'Il Vivaio', which explains the name 'Modello Vivaio' in Italian. It grew out of the meeting between three persons with three different backgrounds and training, but with a common interest in the extraordinary power of emotion, a force which is mysterious and invisible but always present in human relationships. Julie Cunningham Piergrossi was an American-trained occupational therapist who had worked in both the USA and Italy with severely disturbed children. Carolina de Sena Gibertoni, before becoming an occupational therapist, had been an elementary school teacher and was particularly interested in the creativity that was part of the play both with children and those with disabilities. Elisabeth deVerdiere was a French-trained psychologist and psychotherapist. It was this interest in emotions in therapy which led us to the fundamental questions of how occupational therapists can recognise, think about and work with the feelings of their clients and of themselves, while maintaining their basic objective of enabling occupation.

The connection between mind and hands, between emotions, thought and sensory experience, found ample space for study in psychoanalytic theory. We worked in a setting which differed enormously from those of our psychoanalyst

Psychoanalytic Thinking in Occupational Therapy: Symbolic, Relational and Transformative, First Edition.
Lindsey Nicholls, Julie Cunningham Piergrossi, Carolina de Sena Gibertoni and Margaret A. Daniel.
© 2013 John Wiley & Sons, Ltd. Published 2013 by John Wiley & Sons, Ltd.

colleagues and we were determined to maintain the presence of actual doing (not only talking about it) as an essential part of our setting.

We were fortunate to be working in a country where we could apply a psycho-analytic approach to occupational therapy, which was fast disappearing in other parts of the world. In our splendid isolation[1] and without the pressure from the public health service, without the power and demands of the university, without the programmes of an association with rigid rules and regulations, we were able to study, elaborate and apply theories that led to MOVI.

We were continuing with a way of practising occupational therapy learned in the United States (1963–1968) when the psychoanalytic orientation was strong in the profession, following the tradition of Gail Fidler (Fidler and Fidler, 1963) and the Azimas (Azima and Azima, 1959). But while the profession in the rest of the world drew away from psychoanalytic thinking and aimed at shorter, more functional and behavioural interventions, our research began to take on its own identity, looking deeper into the three-way relationship between therapist, patient and 'doing'. Our thinking and practice began to take the shape of a conceptual practice model in Italy around the year 2000, and MOVI with its specific name was presented to the occupational therapy international community at the European Congress in Athens (Cunningham Piergrossi and Gibertoni, 2004) and at the World Federation Congress in Sydney (Cunningham Piergrossi and Gibertoni, 2006).

This chapter will present an overview of the model, describing its basic philoso-phy, its specific characteristics and its seven components, using theoretical concepts and clinical examples.

What is MOVI?

The central element of MOVI is the recognition of the emotions that are in constant movement in the relationship between patient, therapist and 'doing', which are linked in a kind of interdependence (as illustrated in Figure 7.1). All three members of the relationship are considered protagonists, even the 'doing', because each

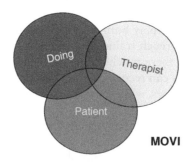

Figure 7.1   The interaction of the three protagonists of the relationship.

---

[1] In Italy the profession of occupational therapy was officially recognised in 1997, and the first university programmes were initiated in 2001.

communicates and transfers something to the other, creating a transference dynamic. In psychoanalytic theory, transference refers to the unconscious links with other relationships in the patient's or therapist's lives, either past or present. (This concept was described more fully in Chapter 3.) MOVI sees this theory as activated also by the doing, which becomes part of the dynamics of the transference. It is interesting to note that MOVI is the only occupational therapy model that includes a theorisation of the presence of the therapist, and it is this fact that gives it its strong relational orientation. Most other models speak of doing or occupation together with the person (client, patient) and the environment. The therapist is obviously present, but not in the dynamics of the theory of therapeutic change (Kielhofner, 2002).

Specific characteristics of MOVI

Considering the example of Matteo, a young boy who had serious emotional disturbance, we can use the intersecting circles to illustrate the concept of inter-dependence. At the end of every therapy session, Matteo frantically grabbed pieces of paper, string and other small objects that attracted his attention, such as a piece of chalk, two peanuts, an eraser, a paintbrush or a cylinder of macaroni. He attached the little package with another string to the leg of the chair where the therapist usually sat, wanting to find it when he returned 2 days later. It was the first thing he looked for when he re-entered the therapy room. Matteo's package expressed his inner world, deprived of an object to hold on to, a sensation of emptiness, maybe the lack of holding (Winnicott, 1971). But it also became a dynamic factor in the relationship with the therapist and expressed his need to be contained, held tightly, attached to something or someone. The therapist reassured him, 'Maybe you are afraid that I will forget about you, that I won't keep you here in my mind. I will be here for you on Thursday at 3 o'clock. I will be here and so will your package.'

The relational experience that moved from Matteo to the therapist and from the therapist to Matteo by means of the package (the transference movements) referred to the link between those three elements that were held together in a kind of interdependence. MOVI theorises transference factors, referring to materials and 'doing' as well as to the people involved. It is a theory that does not exist in psychoanalytic literature, but is introduced and analysed by MOVI because of the presence of objects and materials in the occupational therapy sessions.

Matteo, after 2 years of occupational therapy, no longer made packages, but constructed a wooden track for his toy cars together with his therapist. After every session he put all the little cars in rows attached to each other before he left the therapy room. And that was how they had to remain, attached one to the other until the next therapy session. The slow change in Matteo (who after another year of therapy constructed a garage out of wood, complete with two petrol tanks that pumped fuel to the toy cars that drove up for service) resulted from the inter-connection between the three elements, therapist, patient and doing, thanks to the interactive processes that were slowly created and which were capable of putting the two minds of the therapist–patient couple in contact with each other through doing.

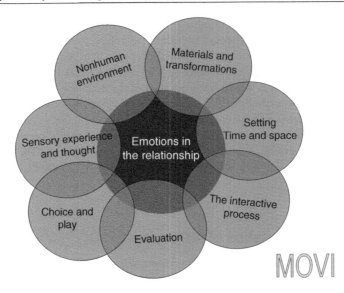

Figure 7.2 Components of MOVI.

The seven intersecting and transparent circles (Figure 7.2) that seem to float around each other like giant soap bubbles contain the seven components of MOVI – the evaluation, the interactive process, the setting (time and space), choice and play, materials and transformations, sensory experience and thought, and the nonhuman environment – and are all connected to the central concept of emotions in the relationship. They are represented as linked circles because none of them stands alone, and all are interconnected. They have no fixed position on the circle and all function simultaneously. If we think about Matteo again, each of these experiences was present in the sequences of the therapeutic session we described, and each was interdependent with the others. There cannot be a setting without an interactive process, a sensory experience that excludes choice, transformations without the nonhuman environment, etc.

The components of MOVI

The seven components of MOVI will now be described, illustrating each one with case studies and theoretical references.

Evaluation

The beginning of the therapeutic encounter is a time for the patient and the therapist to get to know each other. It includes an attentive observation, a precious instrument that remains part of the whole therapeutic process. To really see the patients, listen to their words, see their gestures, their body movements, their glances, their reactions, is a way of holding them in the mind of the occupational therapist. Our fluctuating attention lets us take in the patients in the essence of their way of being with themselves and with others. The capacity for observation that is acquired during the MOVI training becomes a precious instrument for learning to listen without intervening, for being attentive and empathetic towards an emotional resonance that can appear unexpectedly from the inner world of either patient or therapist.

We see the observation as a way of offering respect and creating an atmosphere of containment, an emotional climate that will permit us to identify two different areas of functioning as a basis for a successive therapeutic intervention. One area is that of the patients' external, visible lives, including their occupational histories, their relationships with the human and the nonhuman environment, and their everyday habits, interests and skills. The other area is internal, which means it is linked to fantasies, dreams and desires that can be expressed in the activities that are part of the MOVI evaluation (Gibertoni, 2006a).

The MOVI evaluation can be used with persons of all ages and in all areas of practice.

The use of activities in the evaluation process

The use of activities for getting to know another person comes from the belief that doing is an expression of being. The four activities used routinely in the MOVI assessment process are the creation of a human figure with clay (Shoemyen, 1982), a structured task (puzzle, mosaic, wood), a free painting and a magazine picture collage (Lerner, 1982). With young children between 2 and 9 years of age, symbolic play is considered an important part of the assessment process.

The three brief examples that follow show how activities are used as part of the assessment.

A river, a stick figure and a worm

Anita, aged 22, was in a mental health treatment centre with a diagnosis of schizophrenia. During the occupational therapy evaluation, she immediately communicated her feelings of persecution as she painted herself immersed in a 'river of misery', and at the same time a sense of self as grandiose and omnipotent, represented by a red disk painted over the river that illuminates a centre made up of black circles, which she calls 'all a pile of shit'.

Mauro, 30 years old, well dressed and groomed, demonstrated the contrast between how he presented himself in the interview and how he felt about himself, when he used the clay to produce a human figure without form and a painting that showed just the sketch of a man-like figure that could have been that of a 4-year-old child. The painting depicted a figure with a big round head and stick legs and arms, all out of proportion.

Seven-year-old Jonathan used wood to communicate his fear in the first encounter with the therapist. He used the coping saw to

> cut out a worm with two heads: a worm who lived with his mother and father, only the three of them, without any brothers and sisters (Jonathan actually has a younger brother). He tightly grasped the worm in both hands as if needing to be reassured that the hard material of the wood might be able to protect him outside of the therapy room, and asked to take it away with him.

The relationship in evaluation

From the very first encounter, the patients should be able to perceive, even if at a very primitive level, the therapist's readiness to care about their suffering and not simply to concentrate on repairing a damaged part. They are given the possibility of projecting on to the therapist the image of a person who can be entrusted with all of their malfunctioning parts. Here we are referring to that subtle balance between mind, body and spirit that, due to illness, has disappeared, causing the loss of an integration that had been previously attained. The aim of the initial meeting is to create a positive start through the building of hope and trust in the patient, which implies the possibility of a future restitution of some degree of well-being.

Particular attention in the MOVI evaluation is given to the patient's request for help. Often upon arrival in the therapy room the patients do not have a clear request and they may need help from the therapist to be able to formulate one, to understand that the therapist's role is to accompany them in slowly taking responsibility, able to make requests for themselves. Only in this way can they take up the threads of their lives, within the limits imposed by the illness, but able to make choices in the simple activities of everyday living that will help them to find themselves again in their lives, interrupted by illness or injury.

The therapist's request of the patient is much more subtle: they ask to be able to help, but the patients do not always want to be helped. There are activities and a pleasant room, but the patients may wonder if there is an inner space in the therapist ready to accept their unpredictability – a space to be able to ask oneself what will happen next, without having a preconceived answer ready in one's mind. If therapists limit their requests to help to what they themselves want to give, they also limit the possibility of being open to what the patient brings to the situation, activating emotional and relational states that can compromise arriving at an evaluative truth. At its core, if the MOVI therapists, knowing nothing, are able to stay with the not knowing and begin to construct a story together with their patients, the possibilities are many. As Sandro Bonomo, a Milanese psychoanalyst, puts it:

> *Strong theoretical conceptualization means reading and rereading stories, accompanying stories that have already been written with stories that can be imagined as real (stories and not projects or diagnoses). Not only living in open situations, but refusing the enclosure of descriptions and reconstructions. Living the 'I don't know', because it is in the knowing that the situation becomes unmoveable. Reading a story means constructing it, knowing it, living it.*
>
> (2010, personal communication)

MOVI's *unique contribution to the evaluative process*

Within MOVI, evaluating can be likened to searching for sense in the patient's diverse representational modalities which, alongside the therapist's own emotional resonance, permit the hypothesis of a kind of treatment that will be able to restore rhythm and breath to the new life experience of the patient.

Teaching how to carry out an evaluation that keeps in mind the emotional aspects present in both members of the therapist–patient couple presents some noteworthy difficulties. 'Caring for' patients means taking on some of their emotional pain. MOVI requires clinical therapists to question the use that is made of this pain and what place it has in the evaluation experience.

The close alliance between the science of the mind and the role of emotions and feelings can put us in a circuit of thought nearer to this extraordinary and mysterious mixture that constitutes the essence of what it is to be human. Over the last 30 years, psychoanalysis, which has always considered the central role of emotions in the development of human relationships, has been supported by neurobiological research which affirms that the mind is dependent on cerebral function, but that it develops through relational processes. (These will be explained below when we discuss the interactive process.) If this is true then it is to be taken into account in the important moments of the first encounter with patients in an evaluation, when many different emotions and feelings are active in the reciprocal interaction that constitutes the beginning of every therapeutic and rehabilitative process.

The interactive process

It is research with infants that is beginning to offer an explanation of how emotions and relationships contribute to cognitive function, as well as of how and why relationships can heal later in life (Bruner, 1977; Shaffer, 1977; Brazelton, Koslowski and Main, 1974; Trevarthen, 1977; Stern, 1998).

It has been demonstrated, for example, that human relationships shape the development of the brain in infancy and perhaps even throughout life. In his book *The Developing Mind*, Daniel Siegel (1999) explains: 'Relationship experiences have a dominant influence on the brain because the circuits responsible for social perception are the same as or tightly linked to those that integrate the important functions controlling the creation of meaning, the regulation of bodily states, the modulation of emotion, the organization of memory and the capacity for interpersonal communication' (Siegel, 1999, p. 21).

The data from infant research are valuable for understanding how a relationship is born. These data, together with the psychoanalytic infant observations (see Chapter 12), have helped us to better understand the tight link between interactive processes and mental function at the very dawn of life. The interpersonal events are the necessary key for penetrating the mysteries of the acquisition of mental functions.

Each healthy relationship is made up of many sequences of interaction which comprise the interactive process. The clinical example that follows describes how meaningful relationships with their interactive processes contribute to the growth of mental functions, and demonstrates how in occupational therapy materials and 'doing' can trigger the process.

Occupational therapists enter into people's life experiences, which are made up essentially of simple daily actions within which human relationships and mental functions develop. The dynamic interaction with the environment, which we call occupation, made up of objects, materials, emotions and interpersonal relations, is a fundamental part of learning, of memory and of attention. Our experiences with objects and materials in 'doing' and occupation are precious pieces of the movement between experience, brain and mind (Cunningham Piergrossi and Gibertoni, 2005).

What happens in the therapeutic relationship (according to MOVI) is very similar to what occurs between infants and their mothers or fathers. The therapists are present and accept the patient's self-agency but they are not passive: they interact and add something of their own in an evolving process in which both people proceed and neither remains still. One of the goals of therapy is to use the relationship to nurture the development and use of mental functions which are often either slow to develop or damaged or interrupted by illness or injury. In this model the mental functions which will be put to use are determined by the patient according to his or her choices.

Francesco and the horse

Francesco, a 4-year-old with retarded language development, closed the book of nursery rhymes which his therapist had just read to him and gazed with attention at the book cover on which the head of a horse peeked out of his stall. The therapist asked, 'What name shall we give to this horse? How about Bibo?' Francesco pointed to the horse and murmured something. The therapist continued, 'What does Bibo want? Is he hungry? Maybe he wants some hay? Maybe he wants to go out for a walk?' The therapist added, 'cloc, cloc, cloc' (with her tongue against the roof of her mouth) and with the same rhythm rapped her hand on the table.

Francesco started to rap with his hands on the table. Then he turned, looked at the therapist's dangling leg, moved from her lap down to her ankle and moved his whole body as if riding a horse. The therapist moved her leg together with Francesco and repeated, 'cloc, cloc, cloc'. Francesco rode his horse and laughed happily. Then he got off of the therapist's leg, returned to the book and with his finger pointed at the illustration of the horse, saying, 'Bo-Bo' (instead of Bibo) and 'Ch, ch, ch' (instead of 'cloc'). He looked again at the therapist, pointed his finger at the horse and again repeated 'Bo-bo-ch-ch-ch.'

In a familiar and secure setting (the therapy room), Francesco opened the way (his attention had been attracted to the picture of the horse's head) and the therapist followed his lead, improvising and enlarging the field of interest. The adult spoke clearly with simple rhythms. Her tone of voice and facial expressions communicated admiration, surprise and playful disappointment. The words which accompanied gestures and bodily movements gave significance and made the interaction more alive. The result which was created by both was a well-developed and sophisticated form of play in which Francesco could agree to and organise actions and dialogue together with the therapist. Bruner (1977) speaks of a format, an interaction in which therapist and patient do things together in a stable setting, where the adult creates formats and ritualises them. The 'mentally alive' therapist functioned to keep the attention of Francesco alive, facilitating significant interactional exchanges.

Colours, odours, sounds and various materials all make up an invitation to play, to choose and to contribute to the creation of a familiar and reassuring atmosphere. In this positive setting it is easier for the therapist to create and maintain significant rituals in which the patient can have the confirmation that, with his behaviour, he is able to communicate and to influence the adult's behaviour and obtain a response. Play and choice, which are the privileged modalities of the sessions, often develop spontaneously, linked to improvisations, novelty, surprise and fun – all elements which assume an important role because they induce the creation and preservation of interactive communication.

According to Shaffer (1977), social interaction requires techniques of sequential analysis. If we transfer this idea to therapeutic relationships, it works like this: the patient does something, the therapist responds, the patient responds to this response and so on. This means that the therapist betters the ability to observe what the patient wants to communicate, enters into the sequences which characterise the therapy session, and responds always as part of the sequence of events.

For Francesco the exchanges from the very beginning of the therapy are characterised by significant communication, with a code of meaning which tends to become common for both therapist and patient. The setting for the exchange has a formal structure made up of routine, familiarity and uniformity, a therapeutic process which emerges in every treatment session from situations that are created anew.

The therapeutic process is a combination of an infinite number of fruitful exchanges where the 'mentally alive' occupational therapist will have the role of promoting, organising and maintaining the exchanges using inert materials which become transformed into significant mental material. This means entering into a communicative and emotional exchange with the mind of another by engaging together in meaningful occupations. In the words of Siegel (1999), 'Emotionally meaningful events can enable continued learning from experience throughout the lifespan' (p. 307).

The setting – space and time

The MOVI setting functions as a container, referring to the space used and to the time spent together, and permits the therapist to work with a psychoanalytic form of listening, concentrating without interruptions on the emotions concerning the relationship between therapist, doing and patient. The term 'container' is taken from Wilfred Bion in his book, *Learning from Experience* (1962), a title which in itself is one of the key concepts of our way of carrying out therapy. Bion introduces two key concepts for MOVI, the model of 'container-contained' and maternal 'reverie' (similar to Winnicott's (1971) concept of 'holding'). Bion tells us that at the beginning of life babies do not yet have a thinking apparatus to be able to make sense of the many different sensory experiences that strike them from within and without. They are only able to evacuate the sensations into the mother, whose primary function is that of containing them, making sense of them and finding a response to what the child is feeling. This quality of the mother transmits to the baby the sensation of having a space in her mind, to be thought about and understood.

MOVI transfers the 'reverie' of Bion (1962) and his containment model to every therapeutic situation, both individual and group. In this kind of setting, occupational therapists contain, create a space in their minds for welcoming, thinking about, understanding, making sense and giving a response to the patient or the group, using mind and hands for lessening the chaos of thoughts and feelings which are being expressed both with words and by doing. This whole process is helped by the structure of space and time in which the therapy takes place.

The specific setting for MOVI includes a fixed time schedule with 50-minute sessions for individuals and 1 hour for groups, which in assuming the characteristics of a container guarantees the stability and a space for trust. The real space is defined in a room that contains a small corner kitchen, a woodworking table, an activity table, an easy chair, a small book shelf, a cupboard full of materials for painting, clay, symbolic play, board games, camera, etc. The objects in the cupboard are available for everybody, with the exception of those contained in the single boxes of each patient, which contain objects brought from home or constructed in the therapy room and that are their own property. The materials and tools are respected, and the dangerous ones can be locked away, permitting the therapist to guarantee the safety of the patients. It is the setting with its rules that permits the development of the therapeutic process.

A well-known Milanese psychoanalyst asked us years ago what the first thing that we said to the children was when we were explaining our work with them. Our spontaneous response, 'We will do things together', seemed somewhat inadequate to us beginners. And we were surprised to hear her approve our words: 'They are clear, put the accent on action, the child knows he or she has the possibility of influencing an outcome, that something will happen.'

The MOVI setting can sometimes be difficult to manage, but it is always interesting, lively and unique. It differs from the psychoanalytic setting because its contents invite some form of doing. It does not resemble a school setting because teaching is not its aim. It differs from workshops of painting, ceramics or woodworking because it always proposes a choice of activities and does not necessarily expect creative expression.

Even when treating patients on the hospital wards or at home, remaining true to the principle of psychoanalytic listening, the rules of the setting must be maintained: sessions with a fixed date and time schedule in a defined space and with a clear therapeutic project. A colleague working in a hospital for the elderly managed to maintain the MOVI setting using a suitcase which he brought with him to the wards. It contained small bags of lavender, cinnamon, cloves, knitting and crocheting needles, various types of yarn, handkerchiefs to embroider, mirrors and candy boxes to decorate, small wooden toys to paint, coloured beads to string, postcards to examine and paste, and seeds to plant in little vases. He had created a special setting agreed upon with his patients. One of the activities he carried out with them was the creation of personal picture books, using the postcards of places they knew about together with stories about their lives that he would write under the pictures. The aim of this activity was the recreation of a sense of identity for certain patients who had become depressed and apathetic. They seemed to have lost their vitality and as a result were not moving around the ward, and slowly but surely risked losing their autonomy. The personal book in some cases seemed to bring them back to life.

Choice and play

Play is an example of what we mean by choice because it is self-initiated, original and creative. For this reason 'choice' and 'play' are placed in the same circle in Figure 7.2.

Choice

We work in a room filled with choices, as described above. What really matters is how the therapist participates in the choosing, especially when the patients' choices are not what the therapist would have wanted for them. Getting genuinely close to the patients' internal feelings of terror, to their bizarre, or violent and sadistic, often severely withdrawn choices, and starting to understand them takes years of training. Therapists need to learn how to use the patients' emotions and their own emotions to be able to really help them, to learn how to put words to what is happening and to use thought processes (their own and those of the patients) to talk about the choices and what they mean.

Winnicott (1971) described the psychotherapy situation as taking place in a space that stands between real (external realities) and unreal (internal fantasies), between me and not-me. He called this the intermediate or transitional space and he used the examples of transitional objects of very young children to explain this theory. These are objects which children use, in their own particular way, to bring them closer to their mothers and at the same time to be able to separate from their mothers, to create distance. In this way they gradually learn about who they are as separate persons. An example is the 'nana' of a 2-year-old boy, a doll's blanket that he holds tight when his mother leaves for work, as if he were hugging her. It gives him comfort because it reminds him of his mum, but it is also a reminder that he can get along without her, at least for a short time, that his 'nana' can be controlled by him, that he can choose what to do with it.

MOVI considers occupational therapy as taking place in a kind of intermediate space where the activities and the doing are part of the relationship, just like the transitional objects. It is a space that helps the children to experiment with the real aspects of being, but at the same time permits an exploration of the intangible aspects of living, which spring from their inner world. In Winnicott's (1971) own words, 'an intermediate area of experiencing, to which inner reality and external life both contribute, . . . shall exist as a resting-place for the individual engaged in the perpetual human task of keeping inner and outer reality separate yet interrelated'

(p. 2). In a model based on psychoanalytic theory we look at reality, but we also look at things that are less tangible, such as emotions, fantasies and choices, which would not be possible in the real world where emotions often need to be modulated and behaviour must follow society's rules. We acknowledge and respect the subconscious. We don't specifically teach new abilities, but our clients learn many new ways of being.

Carolina Gibertoni (2006b), in her book on therapeutic cooking, describes how choice can create its own story line and likens the choices linked to doing to Freud's invention of the method of free association. She explains that Freud tells his patients to close their eyes and narrate. They are the ones who choose what to talk about, while the occupational therapist tells patients to open their eyes and choose what to do. The doing becomes a form of narration in its own right. In her words, referring to the activity of cooking:

> *Open your eyes and narrate, say occupational therapists to their patients, immersed in all of the sensory enticements present in our kitchens. And when a portion of that realness becomes usable substance it turns on the mind and begins the story telling. It becomes a story which unwinds and continues through the use of the hands, the materials, the objects and the body. The story helps us to know where the patient is, where the therapist is and what is happening in the 'here and now' of the therapy session. The key to being able to narrate lies in the link between sensory experience and thought, between hands and mind. These then constitute the significance of the tale and the comprehension of the narration.*
>
> (Gibertoni, 2006b, p. 28)

Winnicott (1971) describes severely disturbed persons who, in relationships and relationally, are like young babies. 'They look and they do not see themselves,' he says (p. 112). Here he is referring to the fact that babies need a good-enough mother who reflects back what the baby has communicated to her, who is attuned to her child. It seems that through choice our patients look and see themselves through a good-enough therapist who is able to be attentive and receptive of their choices. What happens is actually very simple and profound: it is in the doing, in participating in chosen occupations in a particular setting and in a therapeutic relationship, that they can begin to see themselves.

MOVI considers the relationship as the focus of the therapeutic process and aims at its construction, attempting to create a space where clients feel contained and protected, and where they are permitted to express their emotions as they can and as they wish. In MOVI the protagonists are always the clients, and the therapist attempts to reach them wherever they may be, offering them the possibility of telling their story through their choices and the transformations that they will succeed in applying to the different materials in the room. When therapists open up their therapy settings for choice, for genuine choice, they must be ready to handle the consequences. 'Genuine' choice means that they cannot foresee what the choice might be and need an open mind to be able to use whatever choice the patient makes as part of the dynamics of the therapeutic relationship and as potential for emotional growth. Genuine choice is not a simple option between two or more alternatives, all of which are ultimately controlled by the therapist. Genuine choice is the invention of something new, using what the therapist puts at their disposition. It is new because it is unpredictable; the therapist doesn't know what will come out, but has a mental space ready to house whatever it might be and to then take it from there.

When we talk to parents about the power of choice in the therapy with their children, they often say, 'Well, what's so great about that? He has his own room filled with things and is always free to choose.' And this is the important realisation: in therapy it is the relationship with the therapist that makes the difference, and the fact that the therapist accepts and thinks about the choices of the child without judging them or attempting to control them.

Marta and the time boundary

Marta, 7 years old, comes into the room and starts asking when it will be time to leave or how much time she has left. Marta loves coming to occupational therapy; she is a creative and talented little girl and uses her time there filling every moment with symbolic or creative play. She is very affectionate with the therapist, but when it is time to leave she begins to change. She is frustrated and angry, begins to whine and to coax, runs and hides in the corner, refuses to leave the room and takes the clay from the container on the table and smears it on her face and arms. Marta says she loves coming to occupational therapy because she can choose what to do. She is the oldest of three children and is very aggressive and difficult to handle at home, has difficulties with her peers and hates school and learning. She has a hard time existing in the present moment, living in the here and now; there is always something else to be wanted. She is never satisfied. In the therapy session the difficulties begin at the moment when the clock says that it is time to go and her possibility of choosing has come to an end. The therapist talks to her about what she is feeling, how hard it is to interrupt what she is doing and how angry she is with the therapist, but it is more than that. The end of every therapy session reminds her of the fact that she cannot always be in control of her life, and that existential fact produces severe anxiety, even in a 7-year-old.

In the course of time Marta's behaviour at home and at school begin to change. Her parents say she is more sure of herself and she has begun to apply her good intelligence to learning. Certainly being able to choose has been very therapeutic for her, but even more, not being able to choose (the limit to the time of the therapy session) has been even more therapeutic. She and the therapist had to work it out together: the wonderful therapist who let her decide what to do during all of the therapy session became the wicked therapist who sent her away. Marta had to learn to put the two together, first of all in the therapist and as a consequence also in herself.

Bion (1962) might have said that Marta was able to experiment a receptive and containing presence and to give meaning to her projective identifications, which in the past had led to feelings of omnipotence. Being able to slowly accept the wicked internal object as a product of her own mind has helped her to tolerate her feelings of frustration and to be more able to learn from experience.

Play

Play is a natural occupation of childhood that continues throughout life in different forms, and by definition cannot be taught or imposed. If a person does not want to play, no one can make him play. Play is a form of intrinsic gratification; it comes from inside and it requires personal choice. All of this is true of adults as well as of children. Adults find pleasure in activities that they themselves choose, that are not imposed by others, and that contain intrinsic gratification. Adults, especially the elderly, do not call their pleasurable activities 'play'. They speak of hobbies or everyday activities like cooking and shopping. To speak of play seems to them to make important activities seem childlike and trivial. In MOVI we continue to use the word 'play' and explain to our adult patients what we mean so that they can start to understand what their significant occupations are in a sphere which is neither work, study nor self-care, but which is equally important for their quality of life.

Giovanna's occupational elegance

At 94 years old, Giovanna is elegant, well dressed and groomed, and very sociable. She especially likes being with others, and enjoys dinner in the residence where she lives. When a recent fall left her with a very painful shoulder injury, she was told by the doctor to stop using her right shoulder for a certain period of time. 'That's impossible for me,' Giovanna explained. 'I need my right hand to get dressed and put on my make-up. Otherwise I can't go to dinner. I lift my right arm with my left one and use it to comb my hair.' The occupational therapist was called because the pain was not diminishing at all and Giovanna was becoming angry and depressed, complaining about the doctor, refusing to cooperate and not accepting a helper in her apartment. The MOVI-trained therapist began by sitting down and having a chat with her client and completely avoiding giving suggestions. She listened and contained Giovanna's pain and fear of losing the ability to 'make herself look good'. For what the therapist began to understand was that Giovanna's true 'play' activity was not just going to dinner; it was dressing well, applying her make-up perfectly, combing her naturally curly hair in a way only she knew how to do. Their first occupational therapy activity was to fashion three different, very elegant slings for her arm of varying colours and materials to match her outfits. It was a fun activity full of memories and lots of looking in the mirror to get just the right 'look'. And as they 'played' together the therapist was also able to talk to her about specific things to do that would help her shoulder to heal faster. These were simple but necessary ideas that would help Giovanna to give her shoulder more rest and that she would be able to understand and accept, such as temporary visits to the hairdresser and learning how to put on a minimum amount of make-up using her left arm and hand.

According to Winnicott (1971), play begins with a child's first choices. He writes about the transitional object (the baby's 'nana') as the child's first real choice. The children by themselves choose what to do with their transitional objects: touch an ear, lip, cheek while holding the blanket, etc., and this is the beginning of play. So it follows that to help children who do not play, who do not know how to play, we need to start from their own choices. Severely emotionally disturbed and autistic children seem unable to play. They don't laugh and enjoy the same things that other children do; they are very serious or sometimes laugh in a bizarre way without seeming to experience pleasure. They are usually unable to have fun with symbolic play, make-believe is impossible, because they use only concrete thought. They learn many things in school and at home, but not how to play.

Autistic children choose sameness. They may be interested briefly in a new object in the room, but they use it in the same repetitive way they use other objects. They seem to search for the sensory aspects of an object: they bite it, tap it on the wall or floor, twirl it, shake it, smell it. The occupational therapist's job using MOVI is to help these children to play, and the only way to do it is by trying to enter into the child's world and start from his or her choices. We try to make the child's choices become something new, something they hadn't foreseen, but something fun and, even more important, something that can be fun together with another person.

Giorgio's game

Giorgio, an autistic boy, one day entered into the therapy room and found a supermarket bag which had not yet been put away. He picked up his favourite stick from the woodworking corner and put the bag over it, twirling it around and listening to the noise of the air on the plastic. He hadn't even looked at the therapist yet. She picked up another stick and deftly took the bag from his, and in twirling it, it flew from her stick into the air. He laughed and caught it on his, and this became a game which went on for some time. An autistic, purely sensory activity had become reciprocal and fun for both. In the next session, she again proposed the bag and stick but the boy was no longer interested. The lesson is a good one: respecting his choices does not mean proposing the same activity again because in doing so the therapist was taking possession of her patient's discovery.

With autistic children we must learn to wait for their timing and to sincerely respect their choices and nourish their creativity.

Managing to uncover the creativity which is in each and every one of our patients is our work as therapists, but of equal importance is uncovering the creativity which is in the therapists themselves. Creativity exists in everybody but sometimes seems invisible because we are searching for something else (Rodari, 1973). When 94-year-old Giovanna's therapist concentrated on inventing elegant slings for her patient's arm, she was not strictly following her activities of daily living (ADL) protocol which called for teaching dressing skills, etc.; she was finding a way of showing her patient that she could still play, even with a temporary disability. If the therapist had been searching only for functional results, her creativity would not have been kindled and her patient would probably not have cooperated, and certainly would not have had a playful experience.

In MOVI the therapist participates in the patient's play. They do things together as part of the setting itself. It might be inventing a story to act out, creating a poem, inventing a new recipe, growing a plant, painting a picture. There are moments when fun becomes the central element of a therapeutic moment.

Francesca's laugh

Francesca, a 6-year-old autistic girl, had been in therapy for 4 years. She seemed to be without thoughts, trapped in her world of tactile and auditory sensations. She did not speak and seemed unable to comprehend language. She never smiled. One day, helping her to put her shoes back on, without thinking or planning, the therapist put one of Francesca's shoes on her own head and asked where the shoe had gone. The little girl looked around and when she saw where it was she looked at the therapist and laughed, clearly amused. The therapist laughed as well. It was an instant of playful contact, providing fun for both that led to a moment of closeness. Entering into a playful relationship with children with severe autism means being ready to act from a preconscious level not mediated by words or even by thoughts.

Materials and transformations

All of the examples of our work with children and adults that make up this chapter contain materials and transformations. During every therapy session our patients cut, pound, paste, cook, eat, play and create. All the things they do to transform materials with their hands and with their minds take on the characteristics of a story where emotions, memories and thoughts travel and intertwine with materials of all shapes, colours and sizes. These then activate new thoughts, new emotions, new memories in a continuous movement between mind and realness (internal fantasy and external reality) (Cunningham Piergrossi and Gibertoni, 1995). During the real transformation of the materials (e.g. the wood with the saw and hammer), a parallel transformation is taking place in the patient's inner world, where the work with the wood is moving memories and emotions, as in the case of Sead.

Sead's home

Sead, a closed and taciturn 15-year-old, chose woodworking as his first activity and was constructing a small house. As he sawed and measured and nailed, he began talking about his biological father. The words seemed intermingled with his actions, as if one depended on the other. He told about how at 7 years old he helped his father make the wooden beds for the caravans where they and their Roma group lived. Sead was very Milanese in his dress and actions, having been in foster care for the past 5 years with an Italian couple who ran a small café bar in the city. The 'house' he was constructing had become the exact replica of his foster father's café bar, but while constructing it, here he was talking about his biological father. Perhaps he was beginning to see himself as belonging to both.

According to MOVI, when Sead began using the wood not only did he transform it into a desired object which united his two 'fathers', but inside himself emotions were solicited which had remained dormant for many years. Thanks to the wood-working and the therapist's interest and containing function, he was able to talk about his confusion and ambivalence, which was particularly important as he entered adolescence. Without the wood the words and the emotions in this very silent boy may not have been expressed. The relationship with the therapist alone might not have been enough, just as the wood-working alone might not have been enough. It was in talking and feeling that Sead was able to arrive at thought and reflection. The therapist helped him to know that he did not have to choose between his two 'fathers' but that he could choose both.

Sensory experience and thought

A key concept of MOVI is that 'doing' can be considered a means for gaining access to the mind. The neurosciences have closely studied the structures of the mind and the link between mind and brain, as well as the importance of social relationships for the development of thought. The ideas and the theoretical aperture that are growing out of this new knowledge, together with Schacter's (1996) studies on memory, have greatly influenced our way of understanding rehabilitation.

The mind uses sensory and bodily organs together with hands to become not only a site of neurons and of neurophysiological processes but a place where emotions are born, memory is stratified, thoughts are animated and the subconscious is hidden. The mind creates a scenario using the senses and decorates it with emotions. In every therapeutic situation, the patients experiment with their senses, creating an exchange between sensory experience and thought, seeing objects and pictures, tasting foods that are salty or sweet, touching surfaces that are smooth or rough. The sensory stimuli are the same for everybody, but are capable of eliciting different memories, unique for each person. They are also capable of creating new memories tied to the here and now of the moment: the nonhuman objects, the human ones, the group, the therapist, the time, the space, the emotions.

Millions of pixels placed in a few square centimetres of brain are lying packed in the dark and the silence of the mind until an odour, a taste, a feeling of warmth, a colour, a sound, takes hold of one or more of them and brings it to the surface, transforming it into an image mysteriously soaked in emotion. The secret lies in trusting the senses soaked in emotion to reach thought processes (Gibertoni 1991).

According to Siegel (1999), the connection with the mind of another person creates a sense of vitality, immediacy and authenticity that can be extremely engaging and stimulating. In these intense moments, in these states of dyadic resonance, we can appreciate how the relationships with others can nurture and care for our minds. For autistic children, sensory experience becomes almost the only means of intervention. Children and therapist jump, sing, play instruments, bake (smelling and tasting) cakes, listen to the echo in a cardboard tube, look at and touch the soap bubbles floating on water. These are the activities that permit the therapist to enter the world of a child who is often closed and isolated in a place which is incomprehensible to others. In the occupational therapy room, they find a person who is interested in their particular sensory way of interacting with the world, trying to make it become relational and playful, an essential step towards the use of symbols and cognitive processes.

It was Giorgio who provided a rare and valuable insight into the autistic world and how occupational therapy can give some respite by using the senses to arrive at thought.

Giorgio's doses of 'doing'

'Dosare gli avvenimenti' (provide the right doses of happenings) were the enigmatic words used by Giorgio for describing our occupational therapy experience, which he had recently concluded. These words were written by Giorgio on an electronic typewriter in the presence of his mother, who had asked him what he had liked doing in occupational therapy because she wanted to continue some of the activities at home. They were using the method of facilitated writing, and his words were strange and seemed to indicate a thought process about his activities that surprised us all. He used very few and isolated spoken words that rarely pertained to what he was doing, and was immersed in a world dominated by the senses. At first, when I thought about what he had written, I thought of 'provide the right doses' as a way of saying 'don't do too much, don't offer too many things, no overload'. But when I reflected more, remembering sessions full of movement, of noises, of 'happenings', it seemed more important to concentrate on the words 'provide the right doses'. Maybe he wanted to say that what he needed was the right dose in the right moment. Defining the 'dose' is certainly a problem for the therapist, who brings something of herself as well as materials to the session, while at the same time encouraging exploration and choice that must come from the patient. Therefore the 'dose' is not a certain quantity, as it is with medicine, but it is an availability of 'medicine-materials-relationship' that is dosed by the therapist and the patient together. Probably his words referred to himself as someone who could choose the right dose of a sensory experience according to his needs during therapy; needs that I could barely sense. I cannot know how conscious he was of my role in permitting and supporting the various doses. But I felt that for him to be in harmony with another person in those moments, to know that the satisfaction of his own needs could be shared and didn't lead only to isolation, could contribute to a sense of self less confused and more complete. The fact that he was able, through the facilitated writing, to put this very complicated idea into words was an indication of his ability to use his senses to arrive at thought.

The nonhuman environment

Harold Searles, an American psychoanalyst, well known for his thinking about schizophrenia, wrote a book entitled *The Nonhuman Environment in Normal Development and in Schizophrenia* (1960). He examined the nonhuman environment (materials, objects, landscapes, trees, houses, rivers, foods and much more) and its psychological meaning, describing a displacement of mental elements belonging to interpersonal relationships on to the nonhuman world. Searles noted the lack of interest among psychoanalysts in the influence of the nonhuman in human well-being and hoped that his work would be an incitement for continuing to explore further an aspect so meaningful in treating mental health problems.

> *Much of the delay in our coming, in the psychoanalytic profession, to a realization of the importance of the nonhuman environment, is attributable to the circumstance that any determined effort to penetrate this area brings up in us the kind of anxiety which, I surmise, we knew all too much of as infants, when the world around us seemed, oftentimes, comprised largely or even wholly of chaotically uncontrollable nonhuman elements.*
> (Searles, 1960, pp. 38–39)

In his work with severely ill psychiatric patients, Searles described their extreme difficulty in separating themselves from the nonhuman environment. They often seemed unable to differentiate human from nonhuman, even during their psychotherapy sessions. One patient with schizophrenia whom we observed in a psychiatric ward had a way of merging with his nonhuman environment which was a clear example of what Searles wrote about. When the nurses would come to give the patient, Ughetto, an injection, he would cover his head with his arms raised up and scream, 'Don't peck my cherries, don't peck my cherries!' Ughetto thought he was a cherry tree, and when doctors or nurses came near he felt like he was being assailed, denuded by a flock of sparrows. 'Don't peck my cherries, go away, leave me alone!' he would yell. His mother said that Ughetto was tormented by a cherry tree growing in their orchard; he was attracted to it and at the same time he feared it and it caused him anguish.

In occupational therapy the nonhuman environment, always present, constitutes the essence of the profession. Occupational therapists are specialists of the non-human aspects of occupations. The application of MOVI underlines the intertwin-ing between human and nonhuman objects in a psychodynamic framework, using the nonhuman for facilitating the quality of the interpersonal exchanges (Gibertoni, 2009).

Often we come into contact with enormous difficulties; we find ourselves confronted with a way of 'doing' of our patients that is crude, disorganised, confused and fragmented. Our task is to consent to them finding some kind of form using their hands and to facilitate the transformation of this material into thoughts, memories and emotions as part of the relationship with the therapist (Gibertoni, 2006b).

Peppino's anchovies

Seventy-year-old Peppino had recently moved for economic rea-sons from a large comfortable apartment to a much smaller place and refused to throw anything away, insisting on bringing every-thing with him, contained in boxes that filled up almost all of the available living space. Peppino had lived alone for many years and alternated moments of psychotic behaviour with others of more mental stability. After moving to his new apartment he began to refuse to eat, to spend as little time as possible at home, wandering aimlessly around the city. He became delusional and one night went to sleep in the bathtub.

Shortly thereafter he was hospitalised for heart problems and when discharged began a home programme of occupational ther-apy with the aim of helping him to create a tie to his new living space and neighbourhood in order to take up again the simple occupations of everyday living that were meaningful for him: food shopping, meal preparation, going to mass, attending a prayer group and going to the movies.

The occupational therapist worked slowly, searching for the subjective experience of Peppino as he began reluctantly to open his boxes and look at his possessions which, with her help, could then be fit somehow into his new habitat. He would laugh and cry without an apparent reason during this process, looking at the objects as if they did not belong to him. The one nonhuman object that finally caused him to pause and reflect was a framed photo of his mother, smiling and happy, who had died many years before. The photo seemed to awaken his memory, and he began to talk about her ways, her cheerfulness and her sense of humour, and most of all to describe in great detail her special way of cooking a delicious plate of fresh Ligurian anchovies.

Peppino together with the therapist decided to dedicate the next therapy session to cooking the special plate of fish and the therapist arrived with the anchovies and other ingredients he had described. Peppino was very alert and, to the therapist's great surprise, began immediately to clean the little fish, throwing away the heads and the insides, filleting each one, opening them like a book and laying them side by side in a round pan, forming a circle of fish. He then added herbs, lemon, oil and bread crumbs and put the pan on the gas fire to cook. As the good smell of fish filled the small kitchen, he looked at them and then at his therapist, hardly believing that he had done it himself. He then set the table for two and went to get his mother's picture and put it at her place: 'Look, do you remember? Today you are eating with me, and I prepared the food myself.' The session was finished, and the therapist left Peppino with his plate of fish and his mother.

The plate of fish, an emotion-filled nonhuman object, became the promoter of a meaningful relationship with the therapist and an investment in Peppino's new home. He began to open the boxes and to 'move in', organising his possessions, buying and cooking his food, and slowly to return to a domestic and social routine that gave him a sense of belonging. The process of weaving nonhuman objects with intrapersonal and interpersonal dynamics began with an object full of affective meaning, the photo of a mother. The process then developed further with the pan full of anchovies, which had become part of a meaningful human occupation.

> *The human being is engaged, throughout his life span, in an unceasing struggle to differentiate himself increasingly fully, not only from his human, but also from this nonhuman environment, while developing, in proportion as he succeeds in these differentiations, an increasingly meaningful relatedness with the latter environment as well as with his fellow human beings.*
> (Searles, 1960, p. 30)

At the beginning of his occupational therapy, Peppino was overwhelmed by his nonhuman surroundings, immersed in them and unable to find himself. After a period of the therapy described, he was able to use the elements from his nonhuman environment linked to emotions, memories and choices to regain a sense of mental stability, a sense of being himself.

Conclusions

MOVI seems to re-awaken psychoanalytic thinking in occupational therapy, which is enormously important to us because it can help our holistic profession to keep hold of a dimension of living which gives depth to who we are as human beings. The contribution of psychoanalytic theories, together with those of developmental psychology, infant observation and the neurosciences, represented an opening and a big step forward in the comprehension of the phenomenology that puts 'doing' in action. Being able to closely examine the meaning of 'doing' created the assumption for the encounter, the link, the relationship, in a mixture of reality, emotions and thought. Doing, another way of conceiving of human occupations, gave us the chance to create the model of occupational therapy that we have described and called MOVI.

References

Azima, H., and Azima, F. (1959) Outline of a dynamic theory of occupational therapy. *American Journal of Occupational Therapy*, 13, 5.

Bion, W. (1962) *Learning from Experience*. London: Heinemann.

Brazelton, T. B., Koslowski, B. and Main, M. (1974) The origins of reciprocity: The early mother–infant interaction. In M. Lewis and L. A. Rosenblum (eds), *The Effect of the Infant on its Caregiver* (pp. 49–76) London: Wiley Interscience.

Bruner, J. (1977) First social interactions and language development. In H. Shaffer (ed.), *The Origin of Human Relations* (pp. 327–347) London: Academic Press.

Cunningham Piergrossi, J., and Gibertoni, C. de Sena (1995) The importance of inner transformation in the activity process. *Occupational Therapy International*, 2 (1), 36–47.

Cunningham Piergrossi, J., and Gibertoni, C. de Sena (2004) The Vivaio model of occupation in the therapeutic relationship. European Congress of Occupational Therapy, Athens.

Cunningham Piergrossi, J., and Gibertoni, C. de Sena (2005) The interactive process and mental functions in occupational therapy. *World Federation of Occupational Therapists Bulletin*, 52, 25–28.

Cunningham Piergrossi J., and Gibertoni, C. de Sena (2006) The Vivaio model of occupation in the therapeutic relationship: The lived experience of five occupation therapists. World Congress of Occupational Therapy, Sydney.

Fidler, G., and Fidler, J. (1963) *Occupational Therapy: A Communication Process in Psychiatry*. New York: Macmillan.

Gibertoni, C. de Sena (1991) Sensi e immagini interne. *Il Ruolo Terapeutico*, 58, 37–39.

Gibertoni, C. de Sena (2006a) La terapia occupazionale e il disagio psichico. In J. Cunningham Piergrossi (ed.), *Essere nel fare: Introduzione alla terapia occupazionale* (pp. 121–151) Milan: Franco Angeli.

Gibertoni, C. de Sena (2006b) *Cibo per pensare: La cucina terapeutica con bambini e adolescenti*. Rome: Borla.

Gibertoni, C. de Sena (2009) Intrecci tra oggetti umani e mondo non umano in un'ottica psicoanalitica, *Giornale Italiano di Terapia Occupazionale*, 3, 59–65.

Kielhofner, G. (2002) *Model of Human Occupation* (3rd edition) Baltimore: Lippincott, Williams and Wilkins.

Lerner, C. (1982) The magazine picture collage. In B. Hemphill (ed.), *The Evaluation Process in Psychiatric Occupational Therapy* (pp. 139–154) Thorofare, NJ: Slack.

Rodari, G. (1973) *Grammatica della fantasia*. Turin: Einaudi.

Schacter, D. (1996) *Searching for Memory: The Brain, the Mind and the Past*. New York: Basic Books.

Searles, H. (1960) *The Nonhuman Environment in Normal Development and in Schizophrenia*. New York: International Universities Press.

Shaffer, H. (1977) The first stages of interactive development. In H. Shaffer (ed.), *The Origin of Human Relations* (pp. 53–67) London: Academic Press.

Shoemyen, C. (1982). 'The Shoemyen battery,' In B. Hemphill (ed.), *The Evaluation Process in Psychiatric Occupational Therapy* (pp. 63–84) Thorofare, NJ: Slack.

Siegel, D. (1999) *The Developing Mind*. New York: Guilford Press.

Stern, D. (1998) *The Interpersonal World of the Infant*. London: Karnac.

Trevarthen, C. (1977) Descriptive analysis of infant communication behaviour. In H. Shaffer (ed.), *The Origin of Human Relations* (pp. 227–270) London: Academic Press.

Winnicott, D. (1971) *Playing and Reality*. New York: Basic Books.

8 Let the Children Speak

Margaret Daniel

This chapter was written as part of a Master's degree in Psychoanalytic Studies at the University of Sheffield and outlines the continuing debate around the contested area of adults recalling experiences of childhood sexual abuse. The feminist movement of the 1970s brought this disputed issue back into the public arena when they suggested that a sexual theory of difference was required to liberate women out of a patriarchal society (Fonagy and Target, 2003). The debate's theoretical roots can be traced back to Sigmund Freud's (1856–1939) concepts of seduction and drive theory, and this will be examined by returning to the early accusations that Freud gave up seduction theory as a way of negating actual sexual abuse. The chapter will focus on the issue of 'false memory' and whether memories can be repressed and retrieved factually. As therapists engaged in therapeutic relationships, occupational therapists need to be alert to the complex needs of people who have survived the trauma of abuse. The two modes of discourse that present the sexual abuse of children as either real or imagined remain poles apart and this chapter will explore the present-day implications for occupational therapists working in the field of adult mental health, counselling and rehabilitation.

Introduction

To understand how the childhood voice of sexual abuse can be heard and contained, we need to consider the conflicting arguments that surround Freud's (1905a) seduction and drive theory. The concerns over what is 'true' continues to affect clinicians when they make contact with the emotional distress of abuse, as it may evoke strong feelings in the therapist of disgust, shock, denial and wishing to attribute blame to the victim. The reason for this is that these stories are difficult to listen to, as well as being difficult to absorb (Draucker, 2006).

Psychoanalytic Thinking in Occupational Therapy: Symbolic, Relational and Transformative, First Edition.
Lindsey Nicholls, Julie Cunningham Piergrossi, Carolina de Sena Gibertoni and Margaret A. Daniel.
© 2013 John Wiley & Sons, Ltd. Published 2013 by John Wiley & Sons, Ltd.

At the start of his psychoanalytic career Sigmund Freud focused his interest, from a male-centred perspective, on the neurotic condition of hysteria, which was seen primarily as a female disorder that lay at the heart of psychoanalysis (Borossa, 2001). He believed that the sufferer's early experiences of external trauma could have an impact on the development of the forming mind (Garland, 1998). Freud began to move away from the suggestible practice of hypnosis and the cathartic method, which induced sleep-like states in patients to relieve them of their hysterical symptoms. Instead he began to focus on what a patient said and did in each of their 50-minute encounters with him. His colleague and mentor Josef Breuer described Freud's method as the 'talking cure'. This was a way of listening to the residue of unconscious material present in the session and moved beyond the use of storytelling (i.e. catharsis) to alleviate distressing symptoms (Freud and Breuer, 1895).

At the beginning of the 1990s professionals working within the field of psycho-therapy and counselling were awakened to a new so-called therapeutically induced (iatrogenic) condition that was spreading from America called 'false memory syndrome' (Brandon, Boakes, Glaser and Green, 1998). Early pseudo-memories of sexual abuse were suddenly emerging in therapy, said to be the result of the therapist's persuasive techniques. Family life was being disrupted and societies, such as Survivors United Network, were established to protect families who were accused of molesting or abusing their children (Merskey, 1998). Celebrities such as the television actress Roseanne Barr Arnold and the daughter of the flamboyant publisher Larry Flint fuelled the publicity by reporting on chat shows their sudden recollections of molestation by their parents (*Independent on Sunday*, 22 February 2004).

From the legal and media professions the finger of blame was pointed at the clinicians, who were accused of using suggestive, hypnotic and regressive techniques (Draucker, 2006). The controversy continues today, as to whether these 'recovered memories' are real or imagined. Alongside these concerns, there were attempts to compartmentalise Freud as a 'recovered memory analyst' (Brandon, Boakes, Glaser and Green, 1998; Crews, 1995; Loftus and Ketcham, 1994). On one side of the argument is the disbelief (or denial) that recovered memories are possible and that they have been blocked through an unconscious process of repression and dissocia-tion. On the other side is the implication, fuelled by our celebrity culture, that it is the clinicians' suggestions that influence their patients' 'recollection' of long-forgotten trauma (DelMonte, 2001).

Brandon, Boakes, Glaser and Green (1998) describe recovered memory as 'the emergence of an apparent recollection of childhood sexual abuse of which the individual had no previous knowledge' (p. 297). The surfacing memories appeared mainly to females in their thirties and forties after many years without any prior awareness. As early as 1932, Aldous Huxley in his futuristic book *A Brave New World* brought to life the harrowing power of suggestibility in his promotion of infantile conditioning as a way to foster a more harmonious society. These 'false memories' are imagined recollections of earlier events that are taken to be true, usually appearing after exposure to suggestive ideas, for example revisiting the believed scene of abuse, or from reading material such as *The Courage to Heal* (Bass and Davis, 1988).

It seemed that society needed someone to blame for its own conflicting and ambivalent attitudes towards childhood sexual abuse. From my clinical experience of working in a sexual trauma clinic, I can recognise that some clients come with the expectation that they will not be believed. At the start of therapy they will be anxious, as they may have been through several other agencies before reaching this service and so relating their story yet again can make it become a presentation detached from emotion to help minimise their distress. However, the retelling of the sensitive story can stir up memories that retraumatise and make the person more disturbed (Spiers, 2001).

Could Freud be responsible?

Freud's work has continued to be placed under intense scrutiny, and invites division and debate where people who take the oppositional positions find it difficult to agree. Freud seemed to mirror this dilemma with his perceived contradictory theories of seduction and drive. Jeffrey Masson (1984), the translator of the Freud/Fliess letters, is one of the main critics of Freud's altering ideas and seems to interpret selectively from Freud's correspondence. His aim was to restore the credibility to Freud's early work on seduction theory and sought proof from Freud's writings to his friend Wilhelm Fliess to re-establish the original theory's importance. In his book *The Assault on Truth*, Masson (1984) challenges Freud's integrity, accusing him of betraying children by altering his theory to suggest that child abuse was only the imaginings of sexual events. Schimek (1986) gave a more grounded and detailed historical account of seduction theory, suggesting that both theories are in dynamic tension as a way to explain and locate neurosis, and thus affirming Freud's change in thinking as not neglectful of outer trauma, as Masson suggests, but a more gradual development of his thinking, locating the impact of trauma from within the inner mind.

More than a century ago Freud (1905a) gave three accounts of 'seduction theory', published in quick succession. In the final account, *The Aetiology of Hysteria* (1896), he presented 18 cases that purported to support his claim that neurosis (i.e. hysteria and obsessional neurosis) was caused by the unconscious memory of infantile sexual trauma. Freud believed the abusers were adults, or older siblings who had been abused themselves (McCullough, 2001). The initial trauma of hysteria was located in early childhood, while the infant was helpless and shocked by the experience. To manage severe trauma, the memories were dissociated, kept separate from the conscious mind, which enabled these incompatible views to exist together (Rycroft, 1995). Obsessional neurosis had a later onset, as it involved the child experiencing aroused pleasure that led to self-reproach (Sulloway, 1979). To defend against the pain of abuse, the memories became actively locked away in the unconscious (i.e. repressed).

Therapy was seen as a way of retrieving these censored memories, inaccessible until resurrected by an event many years later. The surfacing of these repressed memories was problematic due to their delayed onset, so Freud (1896, p. 164) conceived a theory called 'deferred action' as a way of explaining how the traumatic event could resurface at the more physiologically mature point of puberty. For instance, the young person may suddenly recognise the memories following sexual difficulties with a boyfriend or relational problems in marriage or after the birth of a child.

Morvan (part 1)

Morvan was a 39-year-old care worker who was attending occupational therapy on a weekly basis because of her depressive feelings and lack of motivation. Morvan usually smiled a lot but arrived at one of her sessions in a distressed state, saying that she had been disturbed the previous night by a documentary she had watched on television about childhood sexual abuse. She disclosed to the occupational therapist that she had been sexually abused by her uncle, who used to childmind her when her parents went out. The abuse has continued to have an impact on her life, especially during intimacy with her husband and in trusting the people she felt closest to. She felt ashamed and guilty, as her uncle had given her sweets and money, which felt to her like payment for her silence. She had always greatly admired her uncle, who had initially made her feel special by the attention he had given her. Morvan's disclosure made the therapist feel physically uncomfortable, as her own fear had been aroused and she felt as if she wanted to leave the room.

As clinicians we need to consider what we do to manage difficult disclosures such as Morvan's and it is important firstly to address our own beliefs around incest and abuse. As therapists we are not exempt from feeling fear and resorting to defensive forms of activity, to try to relieve the intensity of the feeling arising from imagining the experience, or from identifying with the experience at a conscious and unconscious level. We therefore need to be able to monitor our own feelings so that our fear is low enough to be able to think and catch how we are behaving. Showing the appropriate concern, while remaining empathic and robust enough to hear the account, is essential (Heard, Lake and McCluskey, 2009; Heard, McCluskey and Lake, 2011). Morvan, although distressed, had risked revealing her experience to someone with whom she felt safe enough to do so.

Paradoxically, just as sexual abuse was revealed as a theory about real trauma, Freud began to turn his gaze inwards to an introspective structuring of his theory, by confiding in Fliess, 'I no longer believe in my *neurotica* . . .' (1897, p. 259). Freud's (1905b) dismissal of his patient Dora's 'tales of seduction' seems to support his shift away from the external reality of the experience, towards the inner fantasies of a young girl's sexual desires for her father (Makari, 1998). Out of this change of direction grew the beginnings of psychoanalysis and the development of Freud's drive theory (Dufresne, 2003).

What created this change in direction? Masson (1984) omits to say, but Coiffi (1998) suggests that it was due to pressure from Freud's peers, a dwindling caseload and a growing realisation that his patients and their recollections could be open to suggestion. Sulloway (1979) believed that turning the search for psychic reality inwards brought the concept into safer alignment with Freud's medical peers and away from the unreliability of the unconscious proposed mechanisms of repression and dissociation. From a sociological and feminist perspective (McCluskey and Hooper, 2000; Herman, 1992; Masson, 1984) this had the effect of silencing the child and woman's voice, which was more in keeping with the oppressiveness of the patriarchal era. Freud's move towards the inner fantasies of seduction in his developing concept was seen as desertion rather than development (McCullough, 2001). The child's experience was believed to be fabricated, in keeping with Freud's revised paper published in 1933. In taking this view, Appignanesi and Forrester (2000) believe that Freud drove sexual equality underground, maintaining women as either objects of desire or maternal caregivers.

It is interesting to note that Freud did not choose to call his theory of (external) sexual trauma 'rape', which gave the impression at first glance that victims wishfully wanted to be raped, and in turn downplayed the abuser's role to one of seducer. Forrester (1990) highlights that the word 'rape' is rarely used in psychoanalytic texts due, he believes, to the analyst's reluctance to make moral judgements, preferring the focus instead to be on the person's inner environment and how the unfolding relationship with the therapist may help to unravel past unresolved difficulties.

There was a further inconsistency, in that Freud's retrospective data were not observational and were assumed to be elicited through the 'pressure technique', in which the therapist applied pressure to the patient's forehead to retrieve memories that were not spontaneously forthcoming (Israëls and Schatzman, 1993). These recollections came as a surprise to his mainly female patients, who had no memory of the claimed abuse. Yet in later writings Freud's position shifted to infer that his patients had been misleading him (Freud, 1933). His search for lost memories was centred on trying to understand dreams as a way to reach the unconscious mind. He believed that dreams satisfied past desires and, if they remained unexpressed, could lead to the production of neurotic symptoms: for example, sleepwalking, fainting, paralysis and coughing (Crews 1995). Freud's doubts grew as he began to realise that even in psychosis, repressed memories remain untranslated in the unconscious mind, perhaps impossible to retrieve (McCullough, 2001).

Whether Freud was refining his concept as Sulloway (1979) suggests, or manipulating a career move as Coiffi (1998) believed, Freud, according to Schimek (1986), was building on to his theory of seduction, aware that early memory was unreliable and able to be forced. His attention turned towards the concept that the human mind strives to fulfil a biological and physiological drive. It was not enough to have an outside representation of relationships; it also required an inner sense of relating. External trauma, therefore, became less important to his theory, as sexuality could be aroused from internal built-up tensions (libido) or impulses that led towards a control mechanism which Freud later called the superego (Greenberg and Mitchell, 1983). Historically, sex with a minor was not seen as an aberration (i.e. an immoral or illegal act), but with the rise of the feminist movement in the 1930s the seriousness of the act and its effect on the child victims began to be exposed (Spiers, 2001).

> **Morvan (part 2)**
>
> Morvan's memories from the past had been aroused by a programme on television, and her felt experience of not being protected by her parents could have been re-enacted by the therapist being unwilling to hear her story or acknowledge her distress. Clinicians can often feel ill-equipped to deal with this sensitive area and feel drawn to refer on to other specialist services. However, this has the potential to recreate the original experience of not being listened to and further enforce the person's sense of isolation.

Was mum or dad the culprit?

For Freud's seduction theory to work, it required an anchor to a real early physical event, like the arousing touch of a mother attending to her infant. Yet Freud was aware that not all traumas led to neurosis. He believed a further step was required which led to disharmony, repression and symptom formation. The step into neurosis needed an event to jolt the memories back into awareness and usually happened after puberty (Schimek, 1986).

The father's role as perpetrator further fuelled the public debate, as Freud (1896) made no reference to the father's part in his original theory. According to Schimek (1986), Freud grew to believe that in order for his theory to work the father had to be the original abuser, either factually or in fantasy. Masson (1984) claimed that Freud developed his theory from his patients' disclosures of sexual abuse. However, from this perspective Freud adapted his statement 'almost all my women patients told me that they had been seduced by their father' (Freud, 1933, p. 120) to one which could fit more comfortably into the context of father as seducer in his patients' sexual imaginings.

Certain feminist movements located child abuse in the father's misuse of power (Herman, 1992). However, Millar (1988) contended that their feminist theory required an acknowledgement of the mother's role, in her lack of protection and blindness towards the child's suffering. It took almost another decade for Freud's initial private renunciation of seduction theory to evolve into drive theory, a more interpretative and reconstructive approach that placed a child's sexual feelings within the realms of their inner unconscious phantasy world, rather than focusing on their symptoms and disorders (McCullough, 2001).

In psychoanalysis the word 'phantasy' is used to denote the imaginary places in which a person's desires are activated. This can range from a conscious daydream to the unconscious, darker, hidden desires (Laplanche and Pontalis, 1973, p. 314). Fonagy (1997) points out that there is a delicate overlap between phantasy and reality, as phantasies are always influenced by reality and can coexist in the same time and space.

The language of unnamed emotions

Freud's longstanding friend and colleague Sándor Ferenczi (1873–1933) continued to work with the environmental (i.e. real experience) concept of trauma. Ferenczi maintained his focus on real psychic abuse, in which a parent (sometimes from the same gender) can become more distant and withholding as they struggle to manage their own sexualised feelings, aroused by their maturing child (Symington, 1986). Ferenczi insisted on presenting a paper at the International Psychoanalytic Association entitled 'Confusion of tongues' (1933) and his stance isolated him from Freud and his peers (Balint, 1958). Ferenczi (1933) likened sexuality to a metaphorical language in which adults express passion, unlike the child's language of playful tenderness. If the adult 'dialogue' is too intense or oversteps the boundary (abuse) between an adult and a child, then a language is prematurely and irrevocably inflicted on the child. This new language is often concealed and weighted with adult guilt and shame. It isolates the child, prohibiting him or her from fully living out their childhood with the innocence and tenderness of play that is a rehearsal for what lies ahead (e.g. the exploration of body sensations through games like 'doctors and nurses').

Ferenczi (1932) realised that, like children, his adult patients with neurosis longed to have what was passively beyond their grasp: that is, a good therapeutic experience. For this to happen, trust had to be established in the therapeutic encounter so that the shift into active engagement could take place. The later object-relations theorists Winnicott (1971), Bion (1961) and Bowlby (1988) took up Ferenczi's (1933) belief in a more containing, therapeutic form of maternal love to counterbalance what may have been lost from earlier times. The therapist's approach was through attentive listening, sensitivity and piecing together parts of the trauma without overstepping boundaries. Freud's restrained approach, in contrast, could be perceived as persecutory and withholding, with the potential to recreate the original abuse (1905b). Millar (1988), like Ferenczi, believed that children who gained this premature language of 'passion' could go on to repeat the abuse. However, this did not mean that all victims became abusers, as there was the potential to discover in other significant adults, such as trusted teachers or interested aunts, the experience of appropriate love and tenderness. In therapy there needs to be a way for the therapist to manage their feelings so that they are neither too detached and clinical nor over-intrusive and probing (Reid, Hammersley and Rudegeair, 2007). If the therapist can recognise his or her own discomfort, it may act as a guide to noticing whether the person is disclosing too much, too soon, and being aware that self-disclosure may draw the therapist into defensive activity to manage the unsettling account of the past traumatic event.

Morvan (part 3)

Morvan had a sense of relief in being able to disclose her experience to someone who did not overreact, or give her a feeling of being judged. The therapy session had become a familiar place that felt safe enough for her to share her experience with someone she was beginning to trust.

The occupational therapist sought support from a supervisor who had the appropriate skills and this allowed the therapist to continue to work with Morvan, as she talked about her distressing experience. In supervision the therapist was given the support to focus on the developing relationship she had with Morvan and to consider ways to support and challenge some of Morvan's childhood beliefs.

The occupational therapist did not use leading questions to probe and had a relaxed manner. She let Morvan talk about her difficult feelings of shame and guilt, which stemmed from her childhood belief that she had colluded with her abuser by remaining silent. The therapist helped Morvan to think about how her early experiences were now affecting her present life.

Morvan began to realise that her smile covered up her fear, a familiar way in which she tried to appease her uncle when he had rewarded her silence with sweets. Having someone alongside her to witness her account had been important to Morvan in restoring her well-being.

The malleable mind

The criticism of adult recollections of abuse centred on the issue of repressed memories. These explicit memories can be seen as problematic, as they are required to be retrieved from the unconscious. They surface many years later, triggered by events that echo aspects of the early trauma (recovered memory). However, given that the mind is malleable, 'false memories' can be misconceived as real recollections, especially after exposure to suggestive ideas (Merskey, 1998).

The human mind is complex and does not just replay past experiences. It also reconstructs (biographical memory) to creatively fill in the gaps. Autobiographical memory takes the real event and subjectively reviews and reshapes the experience. It is formed in early childhood and is socially constructed as the personal recollections are revisited. At the same time, few people can recall events before the age of 3, as brain development is not complete (Brandon, Boakes, Glaser and Green, 1998).

Helen's wedding memory

Helen recounted her firm childhood belief that she had been present at her parents' wedding, even though she had not been born until 1 year later. The story only began to alter when she was much older, having spoken to a school friend and hearing for herself how unlikely her recollection sounded. She began to realise that the vividness of the memory came from wedding photographs she had seen as a young child and the veil and tiara she had played with while dressing up, giving a base to her misinformed belief.

Neuroscience is beginning to map out some of these emerging contours in the psychoanalytic landscape, revealing perhaps what Freud was striving to attain: that the relational 'talking cure' he chanced upon was a powerful agent for social and cultural change (Gerhardt, 2004, 2010) and that the parent–baby relationship becomes the human bond which forms the neural connections from which a child's mind emerges (Schore, 2001; Siegel, 1999). Balbernie (2001) also highlights that the inner circuitry of the brain is still forming up to the age of about 3 years and that the connections (synapses) are still malleable and influenced by social experiences. He suggests that repeated childhood maltreatment and neglect can etch its trauma-tising mark on to the matrix of the forming brain.

Where direct and indirect abuse (e.g. neglect) is ongoing, the infant's primitive mental functioning is affected. Balbernie's (2001) research confirms that the brainstem and mid-brain become under-adjusted and affect the child's ability to register danger and alertness to changes in the environment. The repetition of abuse leads to stress responses being laid down in the developing personality and can be at either ends of the continuum, creating hyper-arousal at one end, and dissociation at the other.

The hormone cortisol is secreted at times of trauma (Gerhardt, 2004) and results in lining the area of the right hemisphere, which is involved with implicit memory, so that the initial trauma can be reactivated by other real or imagined situations. The rush of cortisol causes cell loss in the hippocampus, resulting in damage to the areas of learning and explicit memory (Schore, 2001). This explanation, Balbernie (2001) believes, answers why some trauma cannot be recalled but only reconstructed. In serious abuse the suggestion is that 'even though the child will never remember the specific events at any conscious level, his lower limbic system – and the amygdala in particular – does store powerful associations between an emotional state, like fear of pain, and the person or situation that brought it on, associations may be indelible' (Eliot, 2001, p. 298).

Trauma is more than a life event, as it indelibly stamps its life-defining mark on the forming mind and, as Bollas (1987) puts it, the experience becomes an 'unthought known' (p. 111). He is suggesting that unpalatable experiences get stored and carried in an unprocessed way to inform later relationships in a way that has not been thought through, or can later be 'worked through' in a therapeutic containing relationship with a therapist.

The toxic narrative

Memories are vulnerable to suggestion and confabulation can lead to childhood narratives of abuse being seen as true. Childhood abuse, Carter (2000) suggests, engenders intense disagreeable emotions that overload the psychological system through the overstepping of a boundary in a power imbalance, and prematurely awakens the child's sexuality. The boundary turns from a semi-permeable mem-brane into a defensive wall inside which the abusive experiences are imprisoned unconsciously and are only accessible through projective identification, a way in which unacceptable feelings are denied, externalised and felt by another as their own feelings (Laplanche and Pontalis, 1973). Therapy can arouse the lost remember-ings and these can often have a toxic effect on the therapist: for instance, clinicians can find themselves caught up in the reality of the abuse, feeling scape-goated and/or reluctant to listen, for fear of being implicated. In doing so, they can unavoidably recreate the abuse (McCluskey and Hooper, 2000).

Brandon, Boakes, Glaser and Green (1998) take a subjective view of the abusive narrative's incredibility, suggesting that if the story is felt by the therapist to be so unbelievable, 'it did not happen' (p. 304). However, the indescribable experiences of the victims of Fred and Rosemary West (Frost, 2011) could be termed 'unbelievable' and yet they were real and not products of a 'false memory syndrome'. Society remains sceptical as to the plausibility of ritual abuse, putting belief beyond reality, wishing to protect parents and in doing so to silence the child. As Scott (2001) describes, the media narrow their view to the bizarre and sensa-tional without listening to the survivor's story. In 1999 the director Tim Roch brought his first harrowing portrayal of incest and sexual abuse to the public screen in his film *The War Zone* (1999), depicting a family's devastation at the hands of what, on the surface, seemed an attentive and loving father and husband. What the viewer begins to see are glimpses into the hidden world of abuse as the surface veneer is scratched away. The film portrays the son of the family uncovering the disturbing incestuous relationship between his father and older sister and the ripples of pain and destruction that this discovery has on the whole family.

Working within this emotionally demanding area, the therapist has to be receptive to what is happening in the therapeutic dyad, always alert to how feelings can be aroused in both the therapist and patient (transference and countertransference). Fidler and Fidler (1963) recognised that occupational therapists needed to grasp the concept of the unconscious. They believed it could help in understanding the importance of activity-based work as a vehicle for transforming inner thoughts and feelings into visible forms of communication and expression (see Chapter 6).

Transference is a way in which a condensed essence of the person's inner world can be glimpsed (Grant and Crawley, 2002). Freud viewed transference as a way in which unconscious wishes could be displaced from one person (the patient) to another (the analyst). These conscious thoughts were out of context, forgotten recollections from the past, now attributed through a 'false connection' to the analyst (Freud and Breuer, 1895, p. 302). Freud's reductionist view saw this as resistance, where the deep longing to repeat the childhood bond with mother had been turned inwards, producing symptoms to keep feelings at a distance (Laplanche and Pontalis, 1973).

The raw unprocessed material given to the therapist has to be, as Winnicott puts it, psychologically 'held' and, if possible, returned in a more acceptable form (1971, p. 112). Mollon (2000a) describes how these primitive emotions can engender the therapist to enact, or be drawn towards overstepping the patient's defensive bound-ary. This in turn can place the therapist in a position where they may be identified (in taking up a position of rescuing) as the abuser. The therapist then becomes the victim of the patient's retaliation towards the perceived abuser, where actions may be misinterpreted and false memories created. Similar to their childhood experience of abuse, the 'false memories' can silence the therapist, who becomes misheard and misrepresented within the session. This emphasises the importance of regular super-vision as an essential way to detoxify the therapist's emotional debris.

Unexpected feelings

An inexperienced therapist announced to her patient, who had been sexually abused as a child, that her therapy would be ending in 10 weeks' time. The patient quickly became angry, saying to the therapist in a raised voice, 'How could you do this to me. You are the worst abuser of them all!' Shocked by the patient's outburst, the therapist began to strongly feel like an abuser (countertransference).

Mann (1995) believes that from a relational or intersubjective perspective, much activity goes on in therapy outside our awareness, and that therapy may parallel the person's problems in everyday relationships. If unchecked, it can then be acted out, which may hinder progress. Mann considered that we will experience abuse as clinicians which has been turned into activity and that we may become to the client one of their past figures who has let them down. Our task is to contain these feelings without enacting them, which is not always easy. Hoggett (2008) suggests we need to be able to listen to the story and maintain respect in a supportive, companionable way, close and distant at the same time. This may be even harder for a therapist if they themselves are a survivor of abuse (McCluskey, 2011).

Looking beyond the actions

At the start of what should have been Jo's third session, I had inadvertently taken my lunch break and gone to the shops instead. On my return I discovered what I had done. I was caught up in a language of enactment rather than containment. I reflected on what had happened in the previous meetings and was aware of how tired and lifeless I had felt. The third session had been arranged and logged in my diary. This situation was completely out of character for me and my actions were telling me that something was happening that was out of my awareness. I had a long uncomfortable wait until I met with Jo again for her next session. Supervision helped me to see that the massive oversight had the potential to be thought about with Jo, so that what lay behind it could be understood.

I began by introducing the fact that I had not been there for her. Jo passed it off, saying that it was not a problem, but I said that I felt that something important had happened in my not being available to her and wondered if we could look at it in more detail. This opened up how her father had not been there for her as a child, to protect and keep her safe from her brother who used to abuse her. I had been enacting an anguished moment where boundaries were broken and she had been let down and forgotten about by someone who was meant to protect her. This was a powerful physical sharing of a traumatising childhood experience that up until now had not been verbalised. As occupational therapists working with the process of doing, we may find ourselves caught up in the lived reality of the abuse, which can be unconsciously translated into our own defensive behaviour (e.g. lateness, forgetting, etc.) to avoid the felt experience.

As the art psychotherapist Caroline Case (2009) highlights, the person's upset can be internalised by the therapist as a way to restore the cultural norm, and what is being played out in the therapeutic relationship can be overlooked. Perhaps as occupational therapists we might not see ourselves as the experts in this specialist area, and we might focus on the label rather than the person. In referring clients/patients on to other agencies, we may inadvertently be replaying features of the original abuse, where there was no one to listen or give support. When faced with such vulnerability from our clients, fear can infiltrate our work. We can find ourselves moving into defensive ways of operating in order to avoid the pain or discomfort of staying with the experience. Heard, Lake and McCluskey (Heard, Lake and McCluskey, 2009; Heard, McCluskey and Lake, 2011) offer us an understanding of how we repeat relational patterns. They suggest that if a person's careseeking needs have gone unmet, the system of careseeking will be unable to settle (as mentioned in Chapter 5) and this in turn will trigger their self-defence system as a way of managing their distress. For the person trying to give care, it will also be a distressing time as they are unable to ease the careseeker's needs. This response creates mutual distress and suppresses the emotions from a dominant/submissive position where the caregiver is unable to be empathic and supportive.

By being able to listen in an attuned and attentive manner, the therapist is offering him or herself as a witness to the person's painful feelings of hidden shame and guilt. However, the therapist has to consider how robust the person is to continue, and whether the disclosure is at an appropriate point in time, achieving a complex balance between facilitating the disclosure and managing the distress. Their story needs to be respected without the therapist becoming overly intrusive or pulling back too far, leaving the client feeling on their own.

Let the children speak

Mollon draws attention to a concerning pattern which occurs following sexual abuse: that of 'projective annihilation' (2000b, 75). This is a pseudo-projection where someone knowingly undermines another person's character and takes concealed pleasure in their subversive actions (for instance, the Nazis' portrayal of the Jews). In relation to the area of child abuse, Mollon may be suggesting that to maintain a cultural equilibrium it is easier to follow a collective denial of child sexual abuse than to consider its unpalatable existence. This denial can reinforce the primitive childhood fears of not being believed, and escalate into misrepresenting a person as someone other than who they are – a victim.

In 1987 social workers disrupted family life in Cleveland, north-east England, by taking action to protect children from suspected sexual abuse by their fathers. At this time the media fuelled the sensational 'hype' of the accusations and focus was diverted from the shocking reality of abuse, towards the victimisation of the innocent parents (some of whom were abusers). The villains became the persecutory social work department (Levidow, 1989) – a role they are frequently given by the public and media (as in cases such as that of Baby P). The unconscious or suppressed fears of the community were projected away from the family and on to the professionals as a way to resolve (and defend against) their guilt and shame. The abuse was thereby turned around and re-experienced, tarring the somewhat 'heavy handed' social workers as the perpetrators. This could be seen as a projective defence that alleviated the parents who felt threatened by an 'identity of annihilation' but left the social workers burdened by the projections (Levidow, 1989, p. 209).

In 2003, after the death of Victoria Climbié, Lord Laming (a UK Peer) pledged to protect children from abuse and this led to reforms and the creation of a Children's Commissioner to uphold their rights in Parliament, perhaps going some way in giving children a voice (BBC Radio 4, 2004). Sadly, for 8-year-old Victoria, this acknowledgement came too late, as systems became 'repressed' and failed to see her suffering in their poor (defensive) practice and multidisciplinary mis-communication. The professionals involved were blamed publicly, yet Victoria was also let down by the family that was meant to protect her. Her parents had sent her from Africa to stay with a relative in Britain with the hope of giving her a better life. Instead she suffered neglect, abuse and an untimely death at the hands of her entrusted great aunt and her partner. A decade on, sadly the distressing story continues to be replayed with Baby P's suffering at the hands of his mother, her boyfriend and a lodger, again seemingly going unnoticed by the numerous health care services involved in his 'care' (BBC News, 2010).

Fidler and Fidler (1963) would remind us that occupational therapy is a language of communication that fosters a collaborative relationship and where meaning can be sought from what lies behind the activity (p. 17). Activity to the Fidlers was a way to express and demonstrate early life experiences and where, in therapy, conscious and unconscious issues could be recognised. Equally, Mann (1995) would suggest that we need to be alert to what gets jointly constructed, as offering support to someone may place the therapist on the receiving end of the person's projected feelings. Attempts at caregiving may resemble aspects of the early situations that triggered the defensive behaviour, which has brought the client into contact with the health/social care services.

Conclusions

Freud's early discovery of sexual abuse and his altering thoughts on seduction theory, from an outer traumatic experience to an inner incestuous fantasy, continues to fuel the ongoing academic arguments about memory retrieval.

From a clinical perspective, the accusatory finger of blame looming over the therapist's actions in providing support needs to be addressed. This is a complex and sensitive area where strong emotions influence actions. Support structures and governmental policies need to take account of the genuine work that can be done and is being undertaken in many health care settings so as not to drive their experiences underground. However, when accusations are turned towards the professionals (as in the case of Victoria Climbié), it is all too easy to pass the overall accountability on to someone else. Individuals, along with government, need to be responsible, accepting that abuse occurs and that it can also be professionally induced. It seems to me that it is the very nature of the problem of children's sexuality, desires, boundaries and erotic love that makes it so unbearable, and as with Freud's theories, once seen, society finds the reality difficult to endure. The media continue to heighten the profile of abuse and to cast doubts on claims which may or may not be true. However, adults do abuse children and continue to deny it. This premature sexual awakening causes mental health problems and within the clinical world the establishment of the therapeutic frame is essential to give a secure structure from which both reality and fantasy can be explored, and for the working through of these emotional traumas. In caring professions such as occupational therapy the countertransference has to be managed, especially if part of the counter-transference enactment creates an unbearable urge to know more or to disregard what is said as untrue. The child's story, held in the adult, needs to be heard.

References

Appignanesi, L., and Forrester, J. (2000) *Freud's Women*. London: Weidenfeld and Nicolson.

Balbernie, R. (2001) Circuits and circumstances: The neurobiological consequences of early relationship experiences and how they shape later behaviour. *Journal of Child Psychotherapy*, 27 (3), 237–255.

Balint, M. (1958) The three areas of the mind: Theoretical considerations. *International Journal of Psychoanalysis*, 39, 78–79.

Bass, E., and Davis, L. (1988) *The Courage to Heal*. New York: Harper and Row.

BBC News (2010) http://www.bbc.co.uk/news/education-11621391 (accessed 24.7.11).

BBC Radio 4 (2004) *Today*. 4 March.

Bion, W. R. (1961) *Experiences in Groups*. London: Basic Books/Tavistock.

Bollas, C. (1987) *The Shadow of the Object: Psychoanalysis of the Unthought Known*. London: Free Association Books.

Borossa, J. (2001) *Ideas in Psychoanalysis: Hysteria*. Cambridge: Icon.

Bowlby, J. (1988) *A Secure Base: Clinical Applications of Attachment Theory*. London: Routledge.

Brandon, S., Boakes, J., Glaser, D., and Green, R. (1998) Recovered memories of childhood sexual abuse: Implications for clinical practice. *British Journal of Psychiatry*, 172, 296–307.

Carter, F. B. (2000) Relationships as a function of context. In U. McCluskey and C.-A. Hooper (eds), *Psychodynamic Perspectives on Abuse: The Cost of Fear* (pp. 54–66) London: Jessica Kingsley.

Case, C. (2009) Action, enactment and moments of meeting in therapy with children. In D. Mann and V. Cunningham (eds), *The Past in the Present: Therapy Enactments and the Return of Trauma* (pp. 65–85) London: Routledge.

Coiffi, F. (1998) Was Freud a liar? In *Freud and the Question of Pseudoscience* (pp. 199–204) Chicago: Open Court (original work published 1974).

Crews, F. (1995) *The Memory Wars: Freud's Legacy in Dispute*. New York: New York Review.

DelMonte, M. M. (2001) Fact or fantasy? A review of recovered memories of childhood sexual abuse. *Irish Journal of Psychological Medicine*, 18 (3), 99–105.

Draucker, C. B. (2006) *Counselling Survivors of Childhood Sexual Abuse* (3rd edn). London: Sage.

Dufresne, T. (2003) *Killing Freud: Twentieth Century Culture and the Death of Psycho-analysis*. London: Continuum.

Eliot, L. (2001) *Early Intelligence: How the Brain and Mind Develop in the First Years*. London: Penguin.

Ferenczi, S. (1932) Notes and fragments (1930–1932). *International Journal of Psycho-Analysis*, 1949, 30 (4), 240–241.

Ferenczi, S. (1933) Confusion of tongues. In J. M. Masson, *The Assault on Truth: Freud's Suppression of the Seduction Theory*. Harmondsworth: Penguin, 1984.

Fidler, G., and Fidler, J. (1963) *Occupational Therapy: A Communication Process in Psychiatry*. New York: Macmillan.

Fonagy, P. (1997) Panel discussion. In J. Sandler and P. Fonagy (eds), *Recovered Memories of Abuse: True or False?* Madison, CT: International Universities Press.

Fonagy, P., and Target, M. (2003) *Psychoanalytic Theories: Perspectives from Developmental Psychopathology*. London: Whurr.

Forrester, J. (1990) *The Seductions of Psychoanalysis: Freud, Lacan, Derrida*. Cambridge: Cambridge University Press.

Freud, S. (1892–1899) Extracts from the Fliess papers. In *The Standard Edition of the Complete Psychological Work of Sigmund Freud* (Vol. I). London: Hogarth Press.

Freud, S. (1896) Aetiology of hysteria. In *The Standard Edition of the Complete Psychological Work of Sigmund Freud* (Vol. III) London: Hogarth Press. 1978.

Freud, S. (1897) Extracts from the Fliess papers. In *The Standard Edition of the Complete Psychological Work of Sigmund Freud* (Vol. I) London: Hogarth Press. 1978.

Freud, S. (1905a) Three essays on the theory of sexuality. In *The Standard Edition of the Complete Psychological Work of Sigmund Freud* (Vol. VII) London: Hogarth Press. 1978.

Freud, S. (1905b) Fragment of an analysis of a case of hysteria. In *The Standard Edition of the Complete Psychological Work of Sigmund Freud* (Vol. VII) London: Hogarth Press. 1978.

Freud, S. (1933) New introductory lectures on psycho-analysis. In *The Standard Edition of the Complete Psychological Work of Sigmund Freud* (Vol. XXII) London: Hogarth Press. 1978.

Freud, S. and Breuer, J. (1895) *Studies on Hysteria* (Vol. 1). Penguin Freud Library, 1974; reprinted Harmondsworth: Penguin, 1991.

Frost, V. (2011) Writer defends Fred and Rosemary West drama on ITV1. *Guardian*, 2 September, http://www.guardian.co.uk/tv-and-radio/2011/sep/02/writer-defends-itv-fred-west-drama (accessed 29.10.2011).

Garland, G. (1998) *Understanding Trauma: A Psychoanalytical Approach* (2nd edn). London: Karnac.

Gerhardt, S. (2004) *Why Love Matters: How Affection Shapes a Baby's Brain*. London: Routledge.

Gerhardt, S. (2010) *The Selfish Society: How We All Forgot to Love One Another and Made Money Instead*. Cambridge, MA: Simon and Schuster.

Grant, J., and Crawley, J. (2002) *Transference and Projection: Mirrors to the Self*. Buckingham: Open University Press.

Greenberg, J., and Mitchell, A. (1983) *Object Relations in Psychoanalytic Theory*. Cambridge, MA: Harvard University Press.

Heard, D., Lake, B and McCluskey, U. (2009) *Attachment Therapy with Adolescents and Adults: Theory and Practice Post Bowlby*. London: Karnac.

Heard, D., McCluskey, U, and Lake, B. (2011) *Attachment Therapy with Adolescents and Adults: Theory and Practice Post Bowlby*. (2nd edn). London: Karnac.

Herman, L. J. (1992) *Trauma and Recovery: From Domestic Abuse to Political Terror*. London: Pandora.

Hoggett, P. (2008) Relational thinking and welfare practice. In S. Clarke;H. Hahn and P. Hoggett (eds), *Object Relations and Social Relations: The Implication of the Relational Turn in Psychoanalysis* (pp. 65–85) London: Karnac.

Huxley, A. (1932) *A Brave New World* (republished 1977) London: Triad Grafton.

Independent on Sunday (2004) The trouble with Larry. In *The Sunday Review*, 22 February.

Israëls, H., and Schatzman, M. (1993) The seduction theory. *History of Psychiatry*, 4, 23–59.

Kerr, J., and Burchill, C. (1991) Let the children speak. *Simple Minds album Real Life*. London: EMI Publishing.

Laplanche, J., and Pontalis, J. B. (1973) *The Language of Psychoanalysis*. New York: Norton.

Levidow, L. (1989) Witches and seducers: Moral panics for our time. In B. Richards (ed.), *Crisis of the Self: Further Essays on Psychoanalysis and Politics*. London: Free Association Books (pp. 181–215).

Loftus, E. F., and Ketcham, K. (1994) *The Myth of Repressed Memory*. New York: St Martin's Press.

Makari, G. J. (1998) Between seduction and libido: Sigmund Freud's masturbation hypotheses and the realignment of his etiologic thinking, 1897–1905. *Bulletin of the History of Medicine*, 72, 638–662.

Mann, D. (1995) Transference and countertransference issues with sexually abused clients. *Psychodynamic Counselling*, 1 (4), 542–559.

Masson, J. M. (1984) *The Assault on Truth: Freud's Suppression of the Seduction Theory*. Harmondsworth: Penguin.

McCullough, M. (2001) Freud's seduction theory and its rehabilitation: A saga of one mistake after another. *Review of General Psychology*, 5 (1), 3–22.

McCluskey, U. (2011) The therapist as a fear-free caregiver: Supporting change in the dynamic organisation of the self. *Association for University and College Counselling Journal*, May, 12–17.

McCluskey, U., and Hooper, C-A. (eds) (2000) *Psychodynamic Perspectives on Abuse: The Cost of Fear*. New York: Jessica Kingsley.

Merskey, H. (1998) Prevention and management of false memory syndrome. *Advances in Psychiatric Treatment*, 4, 253–262.

Millar, A. (1988) *Thou Shalt Not be Aware: Society's Betrayal of the Child*. London: Virago.

Mollon, P. (2000a) *Postmodern Encounters: Freud and False Memory Syndrome*. Cambridge: Icon.

Mollon, P. (2000b) Is human nature intrinsically abusive? In U. McCluskey and C. A. Hooper (eds), *Psychodynamic Perspectives on Abuse: The Cost of Fear*. London: Jessica Kingsley.

Reid, J., Hammersley, P., and Rudegeair, T. (2007) Why, when and how to ask about childhood abuse. *Advances in Psychiatric Treatment*, 13 (2), 101–110.

Roth, T. (1999) The War Zone (dir. T. Loth). Lot 47 Films.

Rycroft, C. (1995) *Critical Dictionary of Psychoanalysis* (2nd edn). London: Penguin.

Schimek, J. G. (1986) Fact and fantasy in the seduction theory: A historical review. *Journal of the American Psychoanalytic Association*, 35, 937–965.

Schore, A. N. (2001) Minds in the making: Attachment, the self-organising brain, and developmentally-orientated psychotherapy. *British Journal of Psychotherapy*, 17 (3), 299–328.

Scott, S. (2001). Ritual abuse: Listening to survivors. *Young Minds*, 54.

Siegel, D. J. (1999) *The Developing Mind: Towards a Neurobiology of Interpersonal Experience*. New York: Guilford Press.

Spiers, T. (2001) *Trauma: A Practitioner's Guide to Counselling*. Hove: Brunner Routledge.

Sulloway, F. J. (1979) *Freud, Biologist of the Mind: Beyond the Psychoanalytic Legend*. London: Harvard University Press.

Symington, N. (1986) *The Analytic Experience: Lectures from the Tavistock*. London: Free Association Books.

Winnicott, D. W. (1971) *Playing and Reality*. London: Routledge.

9 Working with Difference

Lindsey Nicholls

This chapter was initially written as an essay topic for a Tavistock and University of East London (UK) postgraduate degree in psychoanalytic approaches to working with organisations. Thus the emphasis is on exploring organisational unconscious processes that arise in response to working with clients (patients) who, through the circumstance of their class, race, (dis)ability, gender, age, ethnicity or language, are different from the occupational therapist and/or the social-political 'norm' of that society.

In articulating the complexity which accompanies writing (or talking) about difference, Treacher (2001) wrote:

> It has become commonplace to begin articles on issues of ethnicity with an apology. . . This is also my starting place but I do not want to make an act of contrition about being on uncertain and shaky ground – indeed, one of the arguments of this article is that this is the only place to be. This is not as a place of retreat or resignation but rather, that we have to hold open a space in which I/we know that we do not know entirely what is going on.
>
> (p. 325)

What I think she saying is that talking about difference is never easy, and perhaps, it should never be easy. Her writing captures my own sense of discomfit in trying to write about my professional experiences in this area.

The clinical examples used within this work, described from over 10 years ago, remain relevant today as they explore the way institutions and/or professional organisations (e.g. occupational therapists) can use their empathic understanding of 'difference' to promote the rights of people who may be marginalised by unconscious normative processes used in a society. The work follows Menzies Lyth's (1988) seminal study of (unconscious) social defences used by nurses in acute care hospitals. Her hypothesis was that organisations (or professional groups)

Psychoanalytic Thinking in Occupational Therapy: Symbolic, Relational and Transformative, First Edition.
Lindsey Nicholls, Julie Cunningham Piergrossi, Carolina de Sena Gibertoni and Margaret A. Daniel.
© 2013 John Wiley & Sons, Ltd. Published 2013 by John Wiley & Sons, Ltd.

developed unconscious defences against the powerful emotional feelings that were stirred up by their work. This was especially pertinent for the emotionally demanding care work undertaken by staff with vulnerable patients.

> *Nurses face the reality of suffering and death as few lay people do. Their work involves carrying out tasks which by ordinary standards are distasteful, disgusting and frightening. Intimate physical contact with patients arouses libidinal and erotic wishes that may be difficult to control. The work arouses strong feelings: pity, compassion and love; guilt and anxiety; hatred and resentment of the patients who arouse those feelings; envy of the care they receive.*
>
> (Menzies Lyth, 1988, p. 440)

Menzies Lyth proposed that the defences used by staff groups and/or organisations to protect themselves from overwhelming anxiety became concretised in the form of routines, roles and procedures in that organisation. These structures could potentially support staff in their work but could become unhelpful when they perpetuated a schism between the care work that nurses wanted to do and the work they found themselves told to perform.

> *. . . Menzies Lyth was able to analyse the procedures undertaken in the hospital both as defending the nurses from anxiety and preventing them from progressing beyond it. She identified various practices that in theory were espoused as poor nursing care, but in practice were commonplace, e.g. splitting the nurse from patient, objectifying patients into conditions and ritualising the performance of tasks to avoid the feeling of emotional responsibility for the clients.*
>
> (Nicholls, 2010, p. 58)

This chapter covers unhelpful processes (unconscious defences) that can be used by staff or services to protect themselves from the painful realities of exclusion for clients who are 'different'. It uses four clinical examples to explore ways in which difference is employed or exploited by the organisation, and offers some suggestions as to how occupational therapists can allow themselves to explore their 'cultural incompetence' (Swartz, 2007, p. 36). This notion of never being able to fully know another is helpful in keeping an open dialogue with all clients. Swartz, like Treacher (2001) in the quote that begins this chapter, believes it is more helpful to say we don't know, and we are sure to make mistakes, rather than to assume we can have a full knowledge of another's experience or ready answers for all situations.

> *. . . if we are serious about cultural competence we have to address the related question of our visceral experiences of cultural incompetence – the difficult, secret silences which can become even more shameful and hard to think about in the context of more and more bells and whistles of practice excellence in the field of cultural competence . . . we need to look for the silences around culture and competence, silences which are hard to hear or see . . . We live these silences out but it takes a particular way of looking, and indeed a particular courage to turn these silences into speech.*
>
> (Swartz, 2007, p. 43)

Note: In all the clinical examples used in this chapter, the names and identifying details of the institutions and individuals within them have been altered to protect their anonymity. In order to incorporate the terms used in psychoanalytic and occupational therapy literature, I have chosen to use the terms 'patient' and 'client' interchangeably. I have never thought that one term was better (or less discriminatory) than the other, and I hope that the following clinical vignettes, with their analysis and reflections on the organisational work, will speak for themselves.

Learning from the other

Alan Paton, a South African poet, politician and author, wrote the highly acclaimed novel *Cry, the Beloved Country* in 1948, following his 15-year work role of managing a reformatory for black teenagers who had committed crimes. The narrative, which embodies the pain of a country divided by racial conflict, places in juxtaposition the experiences of two fathers, one white and one black. Their encounter (meeting) produces a deep understanding of each other's experience and, thus, a growth within themselves.

In the story, the black man's (Kumalo's) son had killed the white man's (Jarvis's) son. There is a poignant moment when Jarvis, while sheltering from a rainstorm in Kumalo's church, asks if Kumalo's son (who has been caught and prosecuted) has been given a reprieve from the death sentence. He reads the letter handed to him by Kumalo, who is too overcome to speak, and sees that Kumalo's son has not been pardoned. He says that he does not understand anything of what has occurred and at the same time he also understands it all (Paton, 1988).

It is the capacity both not to understand and to understand completely[1] that is the hypothesis of this chapter. The poetic licence of the novel places these two fathers, through circumstance, to meet each other not only through the trauma of the crime, but in their shared love of a rural village in which Kumalo (a priest) has his church. Their interaction, which shifts between anger, shame, remorse and forgiveness, is a declaration that understanding the 'other' can bring about a change in oneself. It is also my hypothesis that because difference provides us with an 'other', it creates a learning opportunity for any person who wishes to explore their inner processes. This may lead to an understanding that extends beyond oneself to the social and political (emotional) realities of others and thereby may create a climate for partnership and change. Gordon (1993), in writing about racism, stated that it exists in two places at the same time. It is part of the real world, frequently supported by those who have political power and/or social status; and it exists in our internal world. It is this existence in our internal fantasy life that is frequently denied by our more conscious liberal selves.

The following clinical vignettes describe how difference is employed, explored or exploited by organisations. Although each example offers a densely textured account of the dynamics within the organisation, I will be drawing from them only certain aspects of how difference is treated by that particular situation, with

---

[1] I do not believe that any person understands 'completely', but the dramatic language of the novel expresses perhaps the desire to learn and so to understand experiences.

some links to theoretical constructs. 'Difference' covers a wide range of categories, such as race, gender, age, disability, and the roles of 'professional' and 'patient'. The chapter is an attempt to look at some of the consequences and difficulties in working with or ignoring difference as an ongoing dynamic in any organisation.

I do not wish to belie the reality of how difference is imbued with social and political power and that the experience of people who are 'different' can be one of abuse or victimisation. However, the chapter attempts to understand the need for organisations to ignore, exploit or incorporate difference in the service of containing their anxiety. In discussing the 'adoption' of anti-racist policies, Lousada (1994) comments that without the thinking that is required in understanding the dynamics of racism, there may be a temptation to a recourse of moralism, another form of fundamentalism.

> It is precisely the recourse to moralism that has in my view done such a disservice to the cause of anti-racism inasmuch as it obscures the complexities of both the political and the psychological factors that produce racism, and the variety of actions that might be deployed to fight it.
>
> (Lousada, 1994, p. 155)

Employing the split position: evoking admiration and/or fear of contamination

The paranoid schizoid position, as first discussed by Melanie Klein (1882–1960), describes the child's capacity to split objects into 'good' and 'bad'. The child does this in response to their internal experience of discomfort, which is projected outwards and into an object that is then felt by the child to possess those particular feelings.

> Thus the ego has a relationship to two objects; the primary object, the breast being split into two parts, the ideal breast and the persecutory one. . . . . The infant's aim is to try to acquire, to keep inside and to identify with the ideal object, seen as life-giving and protective, and to keep out the bad object and those parts of the self which contain the death instinct.
>
> (Segal, 1988, p. 26)

Many people in times of stress or illness return to a simplistic (fundamentalist) view of the world and use difference as a container for the bad and 'split-off' parts of themselves.

This could be experienced as fearfulness in racial difference, or difference in age, gender or professional position. The feelings of a patient towards hospital staff can mirror the early experiences of the child towards the mother, who is viewed as a split object: that is, not as a whole object.

This was once very clearly expressed to me by a medical doctor and friend (Richard), who was involved in a motor car accident, sustaining an incomplete lesion of his spinal cord, rendering him paralysed from the neck down. He said that in his first few weeks in hospital he thought the nurses had placed extremely heavy blankets on his body that prevented him from moving his limbs. He was convinced they were being deliberately cruel and using these weights to torment him. He said that rationally he knew it was not the case and he was distressed at his paranoid response towards their care; after all, he worked with nurses in his professional role. It seemed to me that immediately following the accident Richard could not allow himself to experience the full impact of his disability, and so he imagined that it was the nurses who were preventing him from moving.

These 'split positions', as Menzies Lyth (1988) had discovered in her work with nurses, can unconsciously become part of the institutional culture of a unit. The benefits and concerns of this ingrained dynamic will be explored with the following clinical example.

Admiration as motivation

The Lavender Project, a drug dependency unit, operates at two levels. There is a 'detoxification' (Fennel) ward where patients are placed on an ever-reducing methadone script until they are drug free (known as 'clean'). This ward is physically adjacent to the recovery (Sage) ward, where patients are no longer using any substances (e.g. diazepam or methadone) and are involved in a group programme which allows for ever-increasing freedom in the community with a view to their returning to their homes or moving on to a further rehabilitation unit. Many of the patients on Sage ward have transferred directly from Fennel ward.

The patients from Fennel ward often say they feel better when they can see the patients from Sage ward, as it gives them an optimistic view of what they will be like. They say that Fennel ward is special because it is 'clean' and that the patients there seem more mature and 'sorted out'. The Fennel ward patients ask for increased contact with Sage ward as they 'look up to them' and they say that speaking with the Sage patients gives them 'hope'.

The organisation of the Lavender Project therefore employs the use of segregation to encourage patients on Fennel ward through their admiration of the 'other(s)' in Sage ward to feel more hopeful. The difference between those clients who are still 'using' (i.e. patients on medication) and those who are 'clean' may help to motivate those on Fennel ward to believe they can survive leaving their drug habit behind. The same admiration for those who have remained 'clean' is seen in the language of Narcotics Anonymous (NA) which speaks about a period of time clean, such as '10 years clean'. The premise in this (NA) recovery model is that drugs are given up *forever more*. Maintaining this fundamentalist (i.e. split) position and institutional separation may benefit patients who have had a chaotic drug using lifestyle and for whom real change would require an abstinence period of many years.

However, in situations where there are clear divisions between 'bad' and 'good', the projected material which has been placed in the other can also be feared. What became apparent to me, in working on the wards, was that many staff viewed the patients in an equally 'split' way, and so feared contamination by the patients. In this NHS-funded unit, the staff had not been recruited from service users or as ex-addicts. The wards often gave explicit messages to the clients that none of the staff had a history of drug using in their backgrounds. The patients often commented on this, saying they admired the staff who were seen as 'normal' but they would equally verbally attack the staff for not understanding what it (addiction) 'feels like'. Although it is not within the scope of this essay to discuss the complex issues around the social inclusion employment policies of many of the health care trusts to employ 'ex-users', I would like to explore a comment made by a staff member from the Lavender Project in the light of the split between patients and staff. The other side of admiration, which could be seen as placing one's good parts in the 'other', is the difficulty in placing one's 'bad' parts in the other, resulting in fear of retaliation or contamination.

> **Fear of contamination**
>
> The nursing staff, who have a small tearoom on Sage ward, wanted to buy a small fridge for their own use. When I suggested, as an interim measure, they put their lunch bags in one of the large fridges in the patients' self-catering kitchen, one nurse, Stella, said she would never do that 'because you never know what they [the patients] would put into it'.

The Lavender Project seemed to operate on maintaining a split position, but in doing so may have created a fear of the 'other', as experienced in the comment of Stella above. Segal (1988) explained, 'The leading anxiety in the paranoid-schizoid position is that the persecutory object or objects will get inside the ego and overwhelm and annihilate both the ideal object and the self' (p. 26).

I wondered if Stella may have been unconsciously re-enacting the split position, which operated on the wards, by concretely responding to the feeling that patients may indeed 'put things into us'. As Ogden (1979) noted in his description of projective identification, clients put their feelings into us as a primitive form of communication, and it is part of the therapist's work to try and understand what these feelings mean. They do this by thinking about their experience with the client. Bion (1962) called this type of thinking 'containment' – taking in and processing primitive experiences in order to make sense of them, even put them into words.

> One major tool at the disposal of the therapist in his efforts at containing his patient's projective identifications is his ability to bring understanding to what he is feeling and to what is occurring between himself and his patient. The therapist's theoretical training, his personal analysis, his experience, his psychological mindedness, and his psychological language can all be brought to bear on the experience he is attempting to understand and contain.
>
> (Ogden, 1979, p. 367)

It seemed that in the Lavender Project this capacity to think about the 'other' was, at times, lost – and as the ward employed the paranoid-schizoid position of functioning, the 'other' was viewed as either 'bad' or 'good' and these differences were encoded in policy and procedure. The fear and anxiety experienced by Stella was expressed as an uncritical thought: in other words, it was an accepted way of viewing and working with the patients. She did not consider that her fear was unfounded; she did not consider that clients could be trusted or enjoyed.

It could be that thinking about the emotional experiences of patients requires an understanding of the introjected material, perhaps feelings of envy, fear or helplessness, as Menzies Lyth (1988) suggested. This thinking about the 'other' would require the staff member to be 'occupied'[2] by the feelings of the patients, described by Bion as the work containment offered to the infant by the mother's capacity for reverie. It may be that this capacity for containment by staff members would have resulted in less dependence on the external boundaries of rule and procedure (e.g. locked doors, urine testing) and more use of therapy groups for exploring the unconscious aspects of the patients' addiction. The Lavender Project made this type of thinking difficult for patients and staff alike as it used the paranoid-schizoid position in the service of a graded (stepped) treatment programme.

Apartheid: the exploitation of difference and the personal price of racism

Holland (1990) in her writing on psychotherapy, oppression and social action asks the reader to consider the fact of racism as a system 'that works' (p. 261). She describes how difference in terms of race has been used by societies as a way of certain groups having access to power, profit and wealth. She states that 'We have to face the fact that racism cannot be eradicated by individual change; it can only be eradicated by in turn eradicating imperialism . . . we must face the fact that racism exists because it works' (Holland, 1990, p. 261).

Apartheid South Africa has symbolised (epitomised) an infamous example of the capacity for a minority group of privileged individuals (white South Africans) to withhold power from a majority population (made of many different racial and ethnic groups in South Africa) by exploiting the notion of racial divisions. As Rustin (1991) wrote: 'race is both an empty category and one of the most destructive and powerful forms of social categorization' (p. 57).

Gordon's (1993) article on 'Psychoanalysis and racism' reinforced this notion of race being an 'empty' category in defining difference. In other words, racial difference is not one that can be based in actual biological or cultural certainty and it may the very nature of this 'empty' category that makes it such an ideal container for split-off parts of the personality. Gordon states that black people in different countries or continents are thought of as being related to each other through the use of uncritical social constructs (e.g. prejudice and power in nation

---

[2] Bion (1962) speaks about the therapist creating an internal space where the introjected material, also known as the transference, can be experienced (and therefore thought about).

states can perpetuate many forms of exclusion) rather than through biological or genetic evidence.

Holland (1990) uses an explanatory model of how the individual patient may be helped through a process of internal recognition of their early life experiences to their social and political reality of oppression and discrimination. She distinguished between loss and expropriation, the former being an internal experience of the loss of loved objects and the latter being what has been taken or stolen from the individual in terms of their position (role) in society.

The help offered to individuals whose symptoms may be a direct result of the reality of their exclusion from society would do little good in offering explanations of their illness if the care environment perpetrated their experience of this schism in treatment. The next organisational example attempts to explore the difficulties when the patient's early life experiences of exclusion and prejudice are echoed in the institution that offered him healing.

Hate in the transference

In 1986 (before the abolishment of the apartheid regime in South Africa), I was working as an occupational therapist in an alcohol addiction treatment unit in Cape Town, South Africa. This hospital had been established as part of the apartheid treatment facilities for the different population groups in the Western Cape. In other words, there was a treatment facility for white patients who abused alcohol, and another separate hospital to treat 'non-white' patients. The hospital, which was located in a 'coloured'[3] area of the city, had a multidisciplinary team in which the only white staff were the consultant doctor and myself. All other staff members, nursing, secretarial, social workers and domestic staff, were 'coloured', Indian and Black. It was common at that time to have white staff work across all the hospitals, but 'coloured', Indian and Black staff could only work in 'coloured' hospitals, thereby with 'non-white' patients.

A patient, Jim McInnes, was admitted for treatment for his alcohol abuse. He was in his mid-forties and had a fair skin, blond hair and blue eyes. He spoke English with an Afrikaans accent,[4] and was very congenial and somewhat subservient in his manner. He stood out in the patient group, as he appeared white next to their brown skins.

[3] The term 'coloured' refers to a racial group who had been given a particular status in South Africa. It may be referred to as 'mixed race' in the UK. The broad population statistics of the Western Cape area in 1986 were approximately 52% 'coloured', 21% white and 27% black. There have been many debates following the change in government in South Africa about the use of the term 'coloured'. This has not to my knowledge been resolved as yet in a country in which privilege was awarded to individuals whose colour defined their status in society.

[4] An accent associated with the 'coloured' group, who were in the majority Afrikaans speaking.

Jim almost immediately formed an intense ambivalent transference towards me, in which he was outwardly appeasing and deferential towards me, but felt I was hypercritical and withholding from him. In a weekly therapy group, following his making a particularly complimentary remark towards my skill as a staff member on the team, I attempted to explore his underlying feelings towards me. This provoked a sudden emotional outpouring in which he stood up, his face contorted with grief and anger, and said I would never understand how much he hated and feared me.

He then told the group of his birth and experience of growing up in a divided (apartheid) land. He had been born as the only son to a Scottish (white) father and a South African ('coloured') mother. On the day of his birth his father went to the registry office and registered him as white. His mother went the following day and registered him as 'coloured'. And so he had been brought up in a 'coloured' area, attending 'coloured' schools and socialising with 'coloured' friends, but he looked white. He described how, when working as a labourer within a group of 'coloured' men, he would be approached as the 'boss' of the group by the foreman of the company, even though he was not the appointed leader. He had become the object of envy for his friends because of the privileges associated with being 'white'. He said when he was drunk and walking down the street, he would feel ashamed when he saw white people because he would feel he had betrayed his/their white skin.[5]

Jim's painful experiences were a result of a multi-layered violence. Explanations of his psychological trauma could be found in the account of the conflict within the parental couple (who would have been denied a legal marriage during their lifetime), and in the early death of his father who had been a distant and critical figure. However, understanding Jim's alcoholism as resulting from inner psychological processes would belie his lived experience of prejudice and social injustice. Jim's story begs us to consider his experience as both an internal conflict and an external reality.

> . . . racism also means psychic injury, a fact that is played down or denied even by anti-racism . . . one does not want to add yet another layer of oppression . . . to the conception of black people as victims. But to pretend that there is no psychic price to be paid for everyday discrimination, abuse and violence – or threat of them – seems to me to be a denial of major proportions . . . we may go so far to say that this silence . . . is itself an injury and an injustice, for it is to deny people a part of their reality, psychic reality.
> (Gordon, 1993, p. 65)

---

[5] The stereotype of the drunk coloured man (a 'klonkie') was in part Jim's way of identifying with his assigned / categorised racial group.

The hospital that offered treatment to Jim in 1986 was not able to consider how it perpetuated the experience of racial hatred and separateness that had been part of his life. It is my belief that in order to engage in some of the thinking about these issues, the staff at that time would have needed to look at their relatedness to each other, as identified by their professional roles and racial groupings. In reflecting on that time, I have wondered about my own difficulty in talking about the pervasive sense of guilt I had as a white therapist working in the 'coloured' hospital. Morgan (1998), in her paper entitled 'Between fear and blindness: The white therapist and the black patient', wrote that pretending there is no emotional dissonance when there is a racial or ethnic difference between the therapist and the client is a form of 'colour blindness' and may represent 'denial' against a painful reality. '[It is] a defence against a complex array of emotions that include anxiety, fear, guilt, shame and envy. No wonder we do our best to avoid the subject' (Morgan, 1998, p. 48).

By avoiding a discussion about our racial difference and thereby keeping the 'other' at a comfortable distance, I may have been defending against my depressive position anxiety. As Kleinian theory states, when an individual moves from a paranoid-schizoid position to a depressive position, they are exposed to their guilt at their destructive impulses and encounter a depressive despair. Added to this was my fear that in talking about my sense of guilt I would expose myself to the full tirade of hate from staff who had been the recipients of such destructive forces throughout their lifetimes: that is, racially oppressive treatment.

> . . . the mourning and pining for the good object felt as lost and destroyed, and guilt, a characteristic depressive experience which arises from the sense that he has lost the good object through his own destructiveness. At the height of his ambivalence he is exposed to depressive despair . . . His pains are further increased by feelings of persecution, partly because at the height of depressive feelings, some regression will recur, in which bad feelings will again be projected and identified with internal persecutors . . .
>
> (Segal, 1988, p. 70)

Since 1988 there have no longer been separate institutions to treat the different racial groups in the Western Cape. But the question in my mind is whether the real inequity in Jim's situation was that he may not have been helped when offered treatment in a facility which represented the internal and external reality of the experiences which led him to abuse alcohol in the first place. Holland (1990) states that the point of psychotherapy (with people who have come from backgrounds of racial discrimination) is to help them separate their 'neurotic hostility towards internalized lost objects/persons from the justifiable rage at oppressive treatment by others in the external world' (p. 267).

Avoiding difference: a need for fusion

Organisations that have been created specifically to offer a service to marginalised groups in society run the risk of denying the difference between society and the client group by 'joining' with the client group. This can be made particularly difficult when staff in the organisation are positively recruited as they are seen as representatives of that difference. When the painfulness of difference cannot be faced, there is a temptation to resort to a manic defence, a denial of the harm experienced by the oppressed individual, and an equally manic reparative drive, which can be omnipotent and essentially patronising in its nature. Lousada (1994), in describing an agency's response to the accusation of racism, writes that it can 'produce a response which, via reaction formation, converts the feelings of persecution (implicit in the accusation) into a thoughtless admiration of the victim . . . Grandiose ambition replaces reality, conflict, discomfort and the modesty of what can be achieved for the client' (p. 157).

The following example comes from a role consultancy (a form of clinical supervision) I undertook at a mental health service established specifically for the needs of deaf clients. There are two illustrations of how this institution managed difference, the one being a manic reparative desire on behalf of the occupational therapist, and the other a fear of difference and need for fusion by an interpreter employed by the service.

> ### Never enough
>
> The occupational therapist, Lucy, did not have a hearing disability and had two years of intensive training in sign language. She was fairly fluent in signing and was both well integrated into the service and respected by her colleagues. Many of the staff (both clinical and clerical) were deaf, and all the meetings were held in sign language. When I visited the unit I was often struck at my sense of being an outsider in a world where people, staff and clients alike, 'spoke' to each other in a language which was both unintelligible to me, and silent.
>
> Lucy was an insightful and sensitive person who was observant of the larger institutional dynamics. She was energetic, conscientious and able to keep modest and achievable goals for her work. However, when returning from a period of leave, she spoke of her great tiredness and difficulty in re-engaging in the unit. She described that when she gets back to work after a break, before she starts to 'cope again', she has a feeling of utter tiredness which comes from the feeling that she can 'not do enough for the clients'. She made an attempt to defend against the feeling and said that 'it always happens when I return from leave and I need to get used to being back'. She then paused and said, 'Sometimes I wonder what I am doing here.'

I wondered if her feeling of tiredness was a result of her getting in touch with the depression that was ever present when working with a group of patients who had a severe disability and whose need to be understood was hampered by both their deafness (lack of speech)[6] and their illness (thought disorder). The positive atmosphere

[6] I am not suggesting that sign language is a deficient language, but that the acquiring of sign language takes significantly longer for the deaf person, and often results in restricted vocational and social choices.

of the institution may have been a manic response to the tremendous difficulty in offering treatment to patients who were already discriminated against in society, whose access to education, work and social engagement was severely restricted.

In Lucy's wondering what she was doing 'here', she may have been trying to make contact with her need to help others, particularly deaf clients, whose experiences did not seem to echo her own life of privilege and purpose. The reparative drive, which is a response to depressive position anxieties, can be the basis for much of the work done with these clients (see Segal, 1988). However Lucy's 'cheerfulness', which following a period of leave threatened to break down, was quickly re-established. Manic reparation (her cheerfulness) denied any anger or guilt in working with these clients.

The atmosphere of the deaf unit was one in which being a deaf person was more highly valued than being a hearing person. Lucy described how, in meetings, hearing people would be criticised for their poor language (signing) skills. It seemed that in this institution you could only be one or the other, but an attempt to be both, a signing hearing person, filled you with a tiredness (sadness) and sense of loss, echoed in Lucy's words: 'I wonder what I am doing here.' It may be this shift from the split (paranoid-schizoid position) to the depressive position of understanding difference that was so hard. In the depressive position, Lucy may have been exposed to her guilt and concern for the lost and damaged phantasy objects, and her response to these feelings may have been to take control and do 'as much as she could', which ironically left her feeling that she could 'never do enough'.

Morgan (1998), in writing of her experience as a white analyst working with a black patient, said the patient, in telling stories of her life, would move between attacks on her therapist's 'whiteness' and self-deprecating remarks about her own 'blackness'. Morgan stated the patient seemed to want her to be black-like-her or remain white and part of the oppressive 'other':

> Was I allied with these white others or would I join with her in her attack, and become black like her? What was not allowed . . . was our difference . . . D could defend herself against the anxiety of longing to become one with me or the terror of expulsion . . . The pain and frustration of me being different and separate from her could be avoided.
> (Morgan, 1998, p. 58)

It may also be that in recognizing difference, the individual, at a psychic level, experiences the painfulness of his first recognition of his difference from his mother, and that a fusion between them is not possible. Basch-Kahre (1984) suggests this may also be the first experience of the oedipal anxiety where the infant recognises that the father (a different face from the mother) offers a real threat to their mother's undivided attention.

When discussing the transference and countertransference that occurs when the patent and analyst are from different sociocultural backgrounds, Basch-Kahre (1984) wrote:

> The analyst may become aware of a feeling of loneliness and helplessness which is cut short by a feeling of anxiety and hostility . . . these are transference and countertransference feelings brought about by the

reactivation of a very early childhood experience, namely the feelings of the eight-month-old baby when confronted with a strange face [the father] . . . [This anxiety] is not merely due to the absence of the mother . . . The father, and later his penis, become symbols . . . They symbolize that the mother has other interests than her baby and that symbiosis with her is impossible.

(Basch-Kahre, 1984, p. 62)

Becoming the 'other'

During a supervision session, Lucy told me that many of the interpreters[7] who worked for the deaf unit were married to deaf partners. She said that some of them, when alone with their partners, would behave as if they were also deaf. For example, they would only answer the door if the light and not the bell were used.

This may be an example of how, in order to avoid the painfulness of separation, and the sense of aloneness, the individual wishes for fusion and then acts as if they are the same as the 'other' (i.e. also deaf).

In these two examples, both Lucy and the interpreter are aware of their difference from the deaf person, but Lucy attempts to remain in touch with her experience of being 'privileged' and pays the price by feeling tired and hopeless at times, whereas the interpreter denies his difference in an attempt to avoid the thinking and experience of inner conflict. It may be this very lack of thinking that can perpetuate discrimination in the realm of diversity.

To think critically one must be able to use aggression to break through the limitations of one's own assumptions or challenge the 'squatting rights' of the colonizer within one's own internal world.

(Hoggett, 1992, p. 29)

In working with institutional change in organisations, the consultant should endeavour to provide a 'thinking space' for the staff group. The challenge of thinking, introducing a third position into the dyad between victim and persecutor, brings with it the territory of uncertainty and ambivalence, and perhaps a real depression (sadness) in the staff for the realities faced by many people with profound and enduring disabilities.

Containing difference: finding oneself in relation to the other

In a paper written for Dr Gordon Lawrence's 60th birthday, entitled 'Satan's return to heaven: The positive aspects of splitting',[8] Evelyn Cleverly sites many

---

[7] These are individuals who are able to hear, speak and sign, and are used to interpret for deaf staff or patients in 'hearing' meetings.

[8] This paper has never been formally published, but seems to resurface in different organisations and psychoanalytic reading groups.

examples of how the mechanism of splitting and projection allows individuals or organisations an opportunity to recognise the split-off part as being in relation to what is held in opposition. She states: 'Integration of a split is not, therefore, concerned with fusion, a blending together, or a kind of coalition; it is concerned with integrity. By that I mean, wholeness discovered and held in paradox through the acceptance and maintenance of coupling among the many, and duality within the one' (Cleverly, 1994, p. 5).

Cleverly (1994) suggests that it is this boundary of a 'thinking space', where the opposites are held in relation to each other, which creates the possibility of a new thought taking place: that is, the birth of a 'third something'. In describing this thinking space, she considers the need for a container that is robust enough to hold the opposites in relation to each other. One such 'container', she suggests, is an intimate relationship, where 'each is certain enough of their own and the other's capacity for recovery' that there can be an environment where 'shared intolerable anxieties can be related to in their projected and introjected form, modified, relinquished and re-owned' (1994, p. 7).

The robustness required of the container resonates with other articles on difference. Morgan (1998) writes about her work with the black patient as needing to be honest and strong enough for a relationship 'that held the possibility of aggression and hate' (p. 60). Lousada (1994) states that what is hard for the 'caring' professions is not the 'failure' of their caring, 'but the anxiety associated with the hateful feelings which are provoked by the client or their condition' (p. 42).

A consultancy offered to an institution (such as a weekly staff group) can provide a container for the clinical multidisciplinary team (MDT) to examine the splits that operate in the organisation and the defences that they may employ to cope with unmanageable (or unconscious) feelings. As Cleverly writes:

> *In my work with organizations I often experience a sense of wonder at the unconscious processes of splitting that develop to protect from, contain and defend against anxiety, and at the same time draw attention (if one is willing to have one's attention drawn) to those very issues that are the source of anxiety, offering them for exploration and naming.*
>
> (Cleverly, 1994, p. 6)

Victims and perpetrators

In 1996 I was asked to run a staff group with an MDT in a small, semi-urban mental hospital. Prior to starting the group, I had met with the managers of the institution and was assured there were no major staff difficulties and the staff had requested a group for 'support'. However, in my first meeting with the MDT staff it transpired that a senior staff member, 'Bill', had recently been investigated for seemingly inappropriate contact with (i.e. touching) some of the young male patients in the hospital.

The staff were extremely distressed and spoke openly about their experience of initially suspecting him of these actions, attempting to report him to the management and their feeling of not being believed. The hospital management, who attended the group on a regular basis, spoke of the measures they had taken to discipline Bill, but were also clear that, although they had taken the matter seriously, he could not be dismissed as there was insufficient evidence.

During this time Bill attended some of the groups[9] and he spoke about his shame concerning his actions. He told the group that he needed help and he had made a commitment to the management to undergo therapy for his problems. After a period of 4 months, he decided to resign because he said he realised that 'doing this type of work made him worse'.

What fascinated me during this long and difficult time was that it was not the expulsion of Bill from the staff group which was the dominant topic of concern, but that individual staff members spoke about their own experience of abuse. After Bill's departure from the organisation, a nursing assistant, Geraldine, said that it had been a particularly painful time for her because, she said, 'My father was like him' (meaning Bill), but she said, 'it wasn't until I started working here that I realised there was help for people like him. I am sad that we [our family] didn't know that he could have been helped.'

The temptation in a situation of such stark conflict would have been to see Bill as bad and the patients as victims, but the group demonstrated a capacity to think about the situation, own their projections and hold the sadness of their experiences. Geraldine's humanity and her concern for the other had impressed me as an example of deeply felt reparative work.

Some further thoughts on working with difference

Gordon (1993), in his thoughtful article 'Souls in armour', says that within the experience of racism, black people do not want white people to love them, but to leave them alone, so they can get on with their lives without having to carry the white person's (unconsciously) projected guilt, shame, envy and anger. He says that the work required of the white person is to learn to love themselves: that is, not project their unwanted parts on to a black person and then crave a relationship with them.

Encountering difference provides us with an opportunity to make contact with our split-off parts, providing we can tolerate the painfulness of incorporating a previously hated aspect of ourselves. However, as Cleverly (1994) points out: 'New discovery and learning, is simultaneously experienced as a "finding" and a "losing", and inevitably demands an ambivalent response. We both welcome new knowledge and resist it to the end' (p. 12).

[9] Because of the ward shift system, Bill, like other staff, could not attend all the groups.

I want to return to the book *Cry, the Beloved Country*, where Jarvis again encounters Kumalo late in the evening on the day Kumalo's son is to be executed for the murder of Jarvis's son. Jarvis asks him where he is going and Kumalo cannot speak because he is too overcome with emotion and mumbles that he is walking to the mountains. Again Jarvis states that he can understand Kumalo's position; he may have said this because he too has lost a son. This empathic reaching out to Kumalo allows him to weep openly in Jarvis's presence. Kumalo then tries to thank him for the money he has donated to rebuild his (Kumalo's) church. Jarvis brushes this halting acknowledgement aside and says he wants to thank Kumalo for helping him out from the darkness of his despair (Paton, 1988). And so Jarvis thanks Kumalo for helping him understand the circumstances of his son's death, the racial tension in the country and mostly himself.

Difference, because it is so, cannot easily be ignored. It demands of us to think about the 'other', and thereby to learn about ourselves. Not to do so, as mentioned earlier in the examples of the staff at Jim's hospital and the nurse on Sage ward, carries the risk of, as Jarvis says, living in darkness. But to engage in thinking about difference exposes the individual to the loss of the familiar, and may be difficult to sustain in a social climate of blame and recrimination. Perhaps in modern (UK) culture the immediacy of trying to establish a cause (i.e. the blameworthy individual or group) for a tragic event can be thought of as a social defence against the overwhelming grief that accompanies a loss, but while the grief and sadness remains unacknowledged, it cannot be worked through.

Conclusions

The price and pain of insight (i.e. critical consciousness) is described by Annette Kuhn (1995), who, emerging from a period in her early life of class discrimination and later educational emancipation, writes about no longer being the 'one' or the 'other'. It may be that this is a position of integration, and within it a capacity for depressive position thinking that allows us to mourn what was not possible and may never be achieved. As Khun (1995) wrote: 'Happily, once embarked upon, there is no end to critical consciousness, to the hunger to learn and understand. Though perhaps for those of us who have learned silence through shame, the hardest thing of all is find a voice; not the voice of the monstrous singular ego, but one that, summoning the resources of the place we came from, can speak with eloquence of, and for, that place' (p. 103). What I think she is saying is that it is this critical awareness that allows us to break through the rhetoric of public opinion and cultural assumptions to become ethically reflexive citizens.

References

Basch-Kahre, E. (1984) On difficulties arising in transference and countertransference when analyst and analysand have different socio-cultural backgrounds. *International Review Psychoanalysis*, 11, 61–67.

Bion, W. R. (1962) *Learning from Experience*. London: Karnac.

Cleverly, E. (1994) Satan's return to heaven: Positive aspects of splitting. Unpublished paper presented to celebrate W. Gordon Lawrence's 60th birthday.

Gordon, P. (1993) Souls in armour: Thoughts on psychoanalysis and racism. *British Journal of Psychotherapy*, 10 (1), 62–82.

Hoggett, P. (1992) *Partisans in an Uncertain World*. London: Free Association Books.

Holland, S. (1990) Psychotherapy, oppression and social action: Gender, race and class in black women's depression (pp. 256–269). In R. Perelberg, and A. Miller (eds), *Gender and Power in Families*. London: Routledge.

Kuhn, A. (1995) *Family Secrets*. London: Verso.

Lousada, J. (1994) Some thoughts on the adoption of anti-racist practice. *Journal of Social Work Practice*, 8 (2), 151–159.

Menzies Lyth, I. (1988) *Containing Anxiety in Institutions*. London: Free Association Books.

Morgan, H. (1998) Between fear and blindness: The white therapist and the black patient. *Journal British Association of Psychotherapy*, 34 (3), 48–61.

Nicholls, L. (2010) 'Putting it into words': A psychoanalytically orientated ethnographic study of hospital based clinical occupational therapy departments in the UK and South Africa. Unpublished PhD thesis, University of the West England, Bristol.

Ogden, T. (1979) On projective identification. *International Journal of Psycho-Analysis*, 60, 357–373.

Paton, A. (1988) *Cry, the Beloved Country*. London: Penguin.

Rustin, M. (1991) *The Good Society and The Inner World*. London: Verso.

Segal, H. (1988) *Introduction to the work of Melanie Klein*. London: Karnac.

Swartz, L. (2007) The virtues of feeling culturally incompetent. *Monash Bioethics Review* 26 (4), 36–46.

Treacher, A. (2001) Ethnicity: Recognition and identification, *Psychoanalytic Studies*, 3 (3), 325–331.

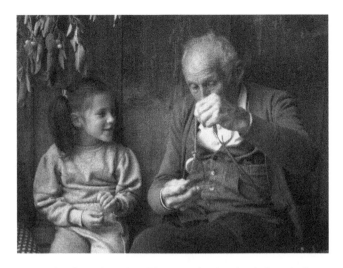

Learning from the other. Photograph taken by J. Cunningham.

Section 3

Further Psychoanalytic Thinking: Research and Training

This final section looks at research methods and projects which acknowledge a conscious and unconscious view of relating to objects (things and people). Chapter 10 describes methods that incorporate psychoanalytic theory, which can assist the researcher in exploring clients' and researchers' experiences (e.g. transference, countertransference and reflexivity). Chapter 11 describes two research projects completed with occupational therapists; the first explores their use of MOVI in clinical work and the second undertakes an analysis of the symbolic use of objects in therapy.

The final two chapters discuss the use of psychoanalytic theory in training courses and supervision. Chapter 12 takes two theoretical roots, psychodrama and infant observation, applying them in undergraduate and postgraduate occupational training courses. Chapter 13 concludes the book by describing a reflexive supervision process that allows for an ever deepening reflection on the conscious and unconscious aspects of what is said and done in the three-way client–therapist–activity relationship.

Psychoanalytic Thinking in Occupational Therapy: Symbolic, Relational and Transformative, First Edition. Lindsey Nicholls, Julie Cunningham Piergrossi, Carolina de Sena Gibertoni and Margaret A. Daniel. © 2013 John Wiley & Sons, Ltd. Published 2013 by John Wiley & Sons, Ltd.

10 Psychoanalytic Thinking in Research

Lindsey Nicholls

This chapter discusses the use of psychoanalysis as a theoretical basis for under-standing a research topic and/or incorporating psychoanalytic methods for gathering information (data/evidence) as part of the research process. Many of the examples are taken from my doctoral study (Nicholls, 2010), which was a psycho-analytically informed ethnographic study of occupational therapists who work in acute medical in-patient settings. To discuss research in these times leads directly to thinking about what is 'evidence' and how it can inform practice.

I would like to start with the quote used by Young (2006), a Dennis Brown prize winner in group analysis for his essay on 'How does group analysis work?':

> *In a speech to the American Academy of Arts and Sciences, 2002 Nobel prize winner for physics, Eric Cornell, asked: 'Why is the sky blue?' I offer two answers (1) The sky is blue because of wavelength dependence of Rayleigh scattering. (2) The sky is blue because blue is the colour God wants it to be . . . this second response does not make God's answer unscientific, just that the methods of science don't speak to that answer . . .*
>
> (p. 477)

In the recent, somewhat persecutory climate of 'evidence-based practice', with its emphasis on the gold standard of randomised control trials (RCTs), I have found it difficult to justify the designing of a study that does not result in a 'scientific' answer. The research I undertook was partly philosophical; it explored the unconscious motives people may have had in becoming occupational therapists. As the social science researcher Hollway (2001) stated:

> *[Evidence-based practice] . . . assumes a seriously reductive definition of what counts as evidence and it claims for scientific evidence an authority, a basis for certainty, which it does not deserve, especially*

Psychoanalytic Thinking in Occupational Therapy: Symbolic, Relational and Transformative, First Edition.
Lindsey Nicholls, Julie Cunningham Piergrossi, Carolina de Sena Gibertoni and Margaret A. Daniel.
© 2013 John Wiley & Sons, Ltd. Published 2013 by John Wiley & Sons, Ltd.

not when applied to human phenomena. The principles of scientific evidence, epitomised in the randomised control trial generally acknowledged to be the 'gold standard' of evidence-based practice, colonise areas of practice which are based on professional caring relationships and threaten to impose reductive and standardised interventions.

(Hollway, 2001, p. 10)

The earlier discussion of why the sky is blue (Young, 2006) may be whimsical, but it seems to capture the spirit of many recent postmodern research methods: that it is not only the question that becomes an ever-deepening iterative reflection (with no rational answer in sight); there needs to be a critical appraisal of the cultural assumptions (i.e. social constructions) behind the stated purpose and methods that are used to gain an understanding of the research subject. I would like to use a simple (personal) example of the problem that positivist research can present when a predetermined set of answers has already been identified, as is the case in some survey designs (or some questioner-led assessment tools). The difficulty with this type of research is that it does not seek to discover, but to confirm what it already views to be true.

Asking questions and knowing the answer

It was mid-morning during the working week; I was at home and had a phone call from a pleasant-sounding woman who said she was a member of a research team undertaking a national study. She asked my permission to interview me and after establishing this was not a ploy to sell me something, I said I was willing to participate. (I was curious about the experience of being a research participant.)

I asked the researcher if she could tell me who had authorised the research. She said she couldn't tell me as it might influence my responses, but I was sure to 'guess' from the first question onwards. I asked what ethical procedure had been used to gain permission for the study and, after a lengthy pause where she consulted her manager, she said she was sure it did have ethical approval but she had only been employed to ask the questions and record my responses, so she asked if we could get started.

She began by asking which of the three UK political parties I supported: Tory, Labour or Liberal Democrats. I replied 'none of them, and so began the difficulty I had with being asked a question in which there was only one answer and no 'other' category where I could say what I had been thinking about. Each question posed, which seemed to emphasise a 'right-wing' political agenda, asked for my opinion on current social welfare policies, the 'problem' of immigration or youth crime. The questions seemed to carry the underlying assumptions that I was dissatisfied with the way things were in the UK, and that I knew who was responsible.[1]

[1] I assumed that I was meant to blame the previous government for its 'woolly liberal-minded policies', which had allowed 'all these foreigners' in. In other words it was these foreigners who were taking 'our' jobs and/or 'stealing' from the overburdened benefit system. The irony in this is that I too am a foreigner.

> The final straw came when I was presented with a list of ten potential 'government tasks' and asked to rank the three most important ones in order. They included limiting immigration, implementing return to work schemes for the unemployed and increasing police presence to combat youth crime. None of the topics matched what I would have said were priorities for the current government, so I asked the researcher (who was becoming more and more apologetic) if I could add to the list she had given me, as it precluded concerns I did have (e.g. the war in Iraq, my opposition to the proposed changes to the NHS, my concern over the marginalisation of youth through the use of terms such as 'feral youth', etc.). 'No,' she said, 'we can't deviate from the list; we can only record the answer you give to those categories.' When I said the list seemed to be a predetermined formula for right-wing conservative thinkers, she whispered, 'I agree.'

I am not suggesting that, as with the example above, all surveys or RCT trials are ethically flawed or carry a politically motivated emphasis with well-crafted predetermined results. The example is to suggest that research into human desires and occupational attitudes needs to have a sufficiently open design to allow participants and researchers to discover new insights that may contribute to our knowledge of being human. This is where psychoanalytic theory can be helpful in its view of people as emotionally complex, paradoxical in their convictions, and capable of deep love and acts of imagination.

The regeneration of psychoanalytic theory in social science

In the last 10 years there has been a resurgence of academic interest in psychoanalysis as a philosophy and/or theory and as a means for gaining knowledge through critical self-reflection (see Clarke, 2006). Social scientists have promoted the use of psychoanalysis as a theory and method in qualitative research projects: notably Hollway, 2001, 2007; Hollway and Jefferson, 2008, 2000; Clarke, 2006; and Hoggett et al., 2006. There has been an interest in (and return to) some of the original thinking and methods used by Freud, who considered that every patient was a new research project.

> *Thus it came about that psycho-analysis, being originally a purely medical technique, was from the first directed towards* **research,**[2] *towards the discovery of causal chains at once far-reaching and recondite . . . Its further course led it away from the study of the somatic determinants of nervous disease . . . it was brought into contact with the mental substance of human lives – the lives not only of the sick, but of the healthy, the normal and the supernormal. It had to deal with emotions and passions, and most of all with*

---

[2] Bold emphasis added.

those which the poets never tire of depicting and celebrating – the emotions of love. It learnt to recognize the power of memories, the unsuspected importance of the years of childhood in shaping the adult, and the strength of wishes, which falsify human judgements and lay down fixed lines for human endeavour.

(Freud, 1919, p. 264)

In many ways it is hard to separate the knowledge (and language) of psychoanalysis from what we 'know' about researching human beings. Kvale (1999) admonishes the scientific (psychology) community for incorporating many of Freud's findings into their everyday language about human nature, but declare his methods as idiosyncratic and theory 'unscientific':

Major parts of psychological knowledge are produced by a method that does not exist in a scientific psychology. General textbooks of scientific psychology today survive parasitically on knowledge produced by a therapeutic method that is denied a scientific status. Two solutions to this paradox appear. One solution would be to censor psychoanalytically produced knowledge, insist that it lies outside the premises of a scientific psychology, and ban it from textbooks of psychological science. An alternative solution would be to regard the psychoanalytical interview as one among many psychological research methods, reflect on its nature, and critically develop its research potentials.

(Kvale, 1999, p. 92)

In 2000 Hollway and Jefferson published their seminal book on *Doing Qualitative Research Differently*. This groundbreaking work has opened the way for research (and researchers) to take into account that human beings have complex emotional lives and that their narratives are layered with consciously constituted narratives and unconscious motivations. I have quoted fairly extensively (below) from an excellent introductory chapter to their work (Hollway and Jefferson, 2008), located in the *Sage Encyclopaedia of Qualitative Research Methods*. In this book they described their disenchantment with certain assumptions in qualitative social research.

. . . generally, face-to-face semi-structured interviewing has become the most common type of qualitative research method used in order to find out about people's experiences in context and the meanings these hold. Considerable effort has been directed to adapting the traditional interview format so that it is adequate to these purposes. But, despite this effort, the idea that an interviewee can 'tell it like it is', that he or she is the incontrovertible expert on his or her own experiences, that respondents are transparent to themselves, still remains the unchallenged starting point for most of this qualitative, interview based research . . . at least one problematic methodological assumption . . . still applies. This is that words mean the same thing to the interviewer and interviewees. In other words, the researchers, in taking this for granted, are still assuming that a shared meaning attaches to words: that the question asked will be the one that is understood.

(Hollway and Jefferson, 2008, p. 298)

Hollway and Jefferson's (2008) hypothesis is that the participant and (to some extent) the researcher are 'defended subjects' (p. 299) and this, unlike the notion of holding something back or keeping secrets, is a normal process in understanding human relationships and eliciting narratives in research. They draw on psycho-analytic theory to explain the layered communication (including conscious and unconscious elements) that is part of any human interaction. In addition to this 'normal' text and subtext in any conversation, research participants may experience a heightened anxiety in relation to the invitation to speak about themselves.

> . . . anxiety is inherent in the human condition, specifically, that threats to the self create anxiety. Defences against such anxiety are mobilised at a largely unconscious level. This idea of a dynamic unconscious which defends against anxiety is seen as a significant influence on people's actions, lives and relations. It means that if memories of events are too anxiety-provoking, they will be either forgotten or recalled in a modified, more acceptable fashion. Defences will affect the meanings that are available in a particular context and how they are conveyed to the listener (who is also a defended subject).
>
> (Hollway and Jefferson, 2008, p. 299)

In a carefully documented account, Hollway and Jefferson (2000, 2008) described how they developed and used the 'free association narrative interview' (2008). This method, which can offer a glimpse into the human experience, aims to elicit real life stories through the use of one or two open-ended questions, which allow the researcher to follow the thread and tone of the participant's story. The quality and depth of the responses by the researcher to what is said (and shared) is a key element to using this method. The researcher needs to have an empathic understanding of what is being said and sensitivity to the context in which it is being shared.

> This approach therefore emphasises the meaning that is created within the research pair and the context within which the account makes sense. It also recognises that the story told is constructed (within the research and interview context) rather than a neutral account of a pre-existing reality.
>
> (Hollway and Jefferson, 2008, p. 303)

Data analysis involves these recorded conversations being transcribed and inter-preted by researcher(s) through a process of writing and reflection. The validity of the results that arise from this method requires that the researcher makes their subjective experience of the participant, topic and context explicit. This sensitively nuanced self-reflection is termed 'reflexivity' (see Finlay, 1998, 2002; Pillow, 2003). The process of self-analysis is potentially exposing and shameful, so it is not easy to do or write about. By using such a reflexive stance in her research, Finlay (1998) writes powerfully about an insight she gained about occupational therapists (and herself, as an occupational therapist) while observing a therapist and client in an acute care setting:

> Although I was supposed only to observe, I found that I could not stop myself becoming involved (by asking the patient questions and even inter-vening at a practical level). When I reflected on my behaviour, I understood that it was due to my active need to be involved, to do something. I also

recognised my own sensitivity as an asthmatic, witnessing someone with breathing problems dying of a lung disease. Once I recognised this, I could then see that the occupational therapist was experiencing similar identifications with some of her other patients.

(Finlay, 1998, p. 454)

An acceptance of psychoanalytic thinking in research allows us to view people as having multiple narratives and unconscious conflicted selves, which do not allow for simple surveys or grand-scale research designs that involve double-blind control groups. But it has provided us with previously 'tried and trusted' routes and/or new methods to gaining knowledge. These are: using observations (Hunt, 1989; Mackenzie and Beecraft, 2004); the clinical interview (see Kvale, 1999) or the free associate narrative interview (Hollway and Jefferson, 2008); and the use of reflexivity where experience becomes the data (Salmon, 2006; Oakley, 2007) or where reflexivity becomes part of the triangulation in the research process (Finlay 1998; Huisman, 2008). Examples of these methods, combined with detailed attention to the social context (i.e. social anthropology), are explored in a book called *Researching beneath the Surface* (Clarke and Hoggett, 2009) and have been termed 'psycho-social research methods'.

In the following section I have drawn on examples from research I undertook into the relational world of occupational therapists who worked in two geographically different acute care settings: South Africa (SA) and the United Kingdom (UK). The procedures used in this study had the interlinking methods of participant observation, interviews and inquiry groups. Throughout this process and encoded in many of the extracts from the data, the reader may recognise the thread of autobiographical reflection. The use of reflexivity, which is central to these qualitative methods, can improve the validity (i.e. authenticity and recognition) of the research.

Psycho-social research methods

The main themes that stand out therefore in psycho-social research are the reflexivity of the researcher; the ability of research to give voice to the research subject rather than a dominant theoretical paradigm; the role of the unconscious in transmitting our ethnic, gendered, and class identities (to name but a few) into the research environment; and finally, again a recognition of the role of the imagination in the research encounter and the way it is used to construct identity and make meaning in people's lives.

(Clarke, 2006, p. 1167)

This quote from Clarke (2006) speaks to the heart of understanding research projects that study people: we live, work and love in a psycho-social world; they are two sides of the same coin. Our belief in the goodness of others (or not) may stem from our early maternal/paternal experiences, but it is the customs and language of our culture, race and gender that affect all that we do and 'see'. I think what Clarke is saying is that we experience ourselves in relation to each other and that understanding occurs in the conscious and unconscious parts of our psycho-social being. This understanding is what we draw upon to make sense of the world and ourselves in it.

An example of this came from my project when, after working and living in the UK for 8 years, I moved back to South Africa. In returning to the 'New South Africa' (i.e. the post-apartheid multicultural society), I realised how much I was still part of an unconscious social world of white dominance. Without this move to a new fieldwork site, I don't think I could have fully appreciated the meaning of Clarke's quote or his work on internal racism (Clarke, 2003). The following autobiographical account, which captures a small event in this process of realisation, became part of the internal scrutiny I had to undertake in order to analyse the data from the South African occupational therapists and clients, the majority of whom were 'black'.[3]

All change

In November 2007 I was sitting with my 83-year-old mother in her room at the Lady Christians Home in Cape Town, South Africa, and reading to her from a book I had brought with me called *The Sunshine Settlers*.[4] This activity could occupy the time we spent together and prevented the repetitive cycle of my mother's questions; she had a progressive dementia and her memory was poor and her attention span limited. She enjoyed being read to and could focus on short, simple stories, and although I had not read the book for many years I remembered it as a series of adventure stories about a man who had attempted to establish a farm in Southern Rhodesia (Zimbabwe) around the time my mother was a young girl – 1930.

Soon after I started reading, I began to struggle as I had to keep substituting words for the ones that were written. I was quite shocked at the racist colonial language of the author and I was acutely aware of the presence of the black nursing staff who were caring for my mother's needs in a way that I had found I could no longer undertake in my own home.

My mother asked me what was wrong, for her sensitivity to the emotional tone of a situation had never diminished. I said that the book had some old-fashioned ideas about black people and I was trying to substitute the words that were written, like 'Kaffir' and 'nigger' as I didn't agree with them. Yes, she said, times have changed and it isn't right to call people those words.

---

[3] The term 'black' is used for its political meaning: that is, it covers all the people who were previously seen as less than 'white'. In this 'black' category are many different tribal, religious, language-speaking and ethnic groups.

[4] Crosbie Garstin, first published in 1935, reprinted 1971.

The vignette described above was one of many occasions when I was confronted with the postcolonial shame I encountered as I saw and felt the legacy of the racially oppressive apartheid past; a past to which I, as a white person, had in so many ways unwittingly contributed, and continued to do so. I frequently found myself out of place (like the example above when I re-read what had been a favourite book of mine) and I would struggle to find other ways of speaking and thinking. This self-scrutiny, undertaken through dream analysis and research supervision, was not comfortable but provided me with a way of re-looking at the data with a lens that included my hidden (i.e. unconsciously defended against) racism.

It also highlights one of difficulties I experienced in writing about research undertaken in a different context from the one that may be familiar to my readers. In reporting on the research, I wanted to provide sufficient contextual detail for the readers to 'hear' and 'feel' the material for themselves. But the words were hard to locate; each word potentially carried a different meaning in the separate contexts (i.e. UK and SA). For example, the word 'indigent' is commonly used in SA to describe 'the poor' and is used as a category (in SA clients' medical folders) to refer to a person who is unable to pay for their treatment. The slippery use of words which can define and/or offend remained difficult for me throughout and I used reflexive accounts in an attempt to locate my understanding (or viewpoint) of the research events and relationships which occurred. As Krog (2009) states in her paper, 'My heart is on my tongue – the untranslated self in a translated world':

> I want to make the point that a narrative can be experienced as discrimina-
> tory and ethically problematic when read through a particular, in this case a
> western, perspective. But the moment there is an attempt to interpret the
> narrative via its embeddedness in an indigenous worldview, it becomes
> breathtakingly ethical, fair and logical.
>
> (Krog, 2009, p. 641)

What I am suggesting is that in using psychoanalytic research methods, a twin focus needs to be kept: on what is being said (or done) by the participant; and on the internal dialogue and associations that are part of the observer's experience. When both are presented, the reader is able to assess for themselves if the insights that have arisen from the data analysis (overall study) have validity. In other words, the group of research participants would recognise the description of their experience as being true (congruent with how they feel and think) and the reader is able to see explicit examples of how the conclusions were reached (transparency and authenticity).

Participant observation: creating an internal map of psycho-social work

Participant observation comes from a long tradition of ethnographic fieldwork studies (Hunt, 1989; Hammersley, 1992; Hammersley and Atkinson, 1995; Gilbert, 2001). As psychoanalytic thinking began to be incorporated into this ethnographic stance, Ester Bick's (1901–1983) method of 'infant observation' (Bick, 1964) drew the researcher into making detailed recordings of every moment of what they observed; externally and internally (i.e. reflections and associations). There are many examples of this type of research (e.g. Hollway, 2007; Urwin, 2007; Skogstad, 2004; Hinshelwood, 2002; Rustin, 1989) but none captured more eloquently than in Mackenzie and Beecraft's (2004) article on observations undertaken in older adult care facilities. Observations cannot only be an account of factual occurrences, because what is 'seen' may be affected by what the observer expects to see (or can cope with seeing, or judges from their social-political worldview), while participants may be affected by the act of being observed.

To create an awareness of the work undertaken by occupational therapists, I spent several periods immersed in observations of their work: with clients, in meetings and at the team base. This was to familiarise myself with the environment by observing the occupational therapists' interactions with clients (including their emotional engagement and tasks performed) and reflecting on my feelings in response to these events. This period gave me an internal landscape of the work and became crucial in developing relationships with the participants. It was similar to Hunt's (1989) description of the importance of the informal time she spent with 'rookies' and officers in the study she undertook on police culture. Hunt stated:

> The initial period of participant observation allows for the development of sufficient rapport with subjects to ensure their trust and cooperation. It also ensures that researchers are familiar enough with the world of research to formulate culturally relevant questions based on their understanding of native meaning structures rather than a priori assumptions.
>
> (Hunt, 1989, p. 13)

After each observation, I wrote detailed notes and reflected on what I had seen and felt. I was able to refer to these notes later in the free associative narrative interviews (FANIs) with the occupational therapists. Thus the recorded events involved a mixture of external actions and internal emotions and associations, similar to the tradition of infant observation that Bick (1964) had required.

The following example is taken from an observation period I had undertaken in the UK acute medical wards. I was often amazed at how busy and noisy the hospital was. There was a continuous movement of staff walking from one place to another, unloading trolleys, pushing clients in wheelchairs and working at reception desks or cleaning ward floors. Clients sometimes seemed out of place in all this busyness because they were static (often in beds connected to monitors) or on trolleys or wheelchairs being taken from place to place. There seemed to be more staff than clients in wards or corridors, and much of the staff time was spent in talking to each other about the clients. This was to confirm and communicate information about a client or a brief reflection on an event concerning a client.

Emotional management in a busy environment

I heard the ward sister talking to a junior nurse. She said a patient (Jake) had died, and added, in a hushed, lowered tone, that he had died from an overdose. She seemed upset and looked distracted. She said Jake had come to the ward the previous week to say hello;

she said they had all worked so hard on him. They had received a call from the drug and alcohol liaison nurse to say he had died.

While this was taking place, I was aware (again) of how busy wards were. Next to the nurses' station a porter was unloading boxes into a store room, there was a cleaner who was moving down the ward with a mop and bucket, and the physiotherapist came behind the nurses' desk to look at some folders and spoke to the occupational therapists, who were writing in the patient's notes. Behind the nurses' station, two doctors were using computer terminals to write their notes. I was watching the number of interactions at any one time that were superimposed on the discussion about the patient who had killed himself. An older woman approached me to ask if she could visit her friend on the ward. I directed her to the ward clerk, who told her which room her friend was in.

From the above observation I realised that there was little time to absorb sad news or find a space in which to retreat to grieve a loss. The constant stream of people and requests would interrupt any emotional response to sad news or a poignant event.

The 'Bick' (1964) method of infant observation encouraged the trainee therapist to observe the details of events which took place between the child and their mother (or father/caregivers), including an uncensored description of their thoughts and feelings during these observations. These were transcribed into detailed field notes that were used in seminar group discussions for further analysis. In this way the researcher relied on their internal experiences (of identification with the subject or experience of projective identification from the subject) to understand the unconscious communication which took place between mother and child.

In a similar fashion, the experience of the fieldwork in my research with occupational therapists provided me with an internal awareness of the emotional work undertaken by the therapists. Some of this awareness was in thoughts, questions, dream images or associations with events in my life. The creation of these internal images and reflections was important in engaging in the next stage of the study, the interview. An unexpected and important aspect of the observation period was that it provided a relational link between me and the therapists whom I followed around as they undertook their daily work. The occupational therapists were aware I had witnessed their work, often 'warts and all', and this allowed them to speak about their fears, frustrations and disappointments, as demonstrated in the following example.

From my first contact with the large London hospital where the occupational therapy department was based, I was struck at how the clients – elderly, frail and in hospital pyjamas – were the ones who looked out of place in the new buildings. The atmosphere of busyness, social interaction and administrative processes seemed to deny the reality of the clients' vulnerability. In going on to the wards and witnessing (at close range) physically frail clients, I realised that not all of them recovered in hospital; some died.

This contrast between the staff activity and the immobility of illness was reflected in the difference between many of the occupational therapists and their clients. The research participants were young and female, and often had an energetic walk and purposeful way of addressing clients (e.g. asking them about their home circumstances or to demonstrate their self-care routines). It seemed as if the occupational therapists did not notice that their clients were much older men who may have found these requests, especially as they were made by a young woman, humiliating.

During an observation period with Caitlyn (a newly qualified therapist), an older male client became angry with her as he said she had not given him sufficient advice and help with his return home. His anger seemed to be a fear of returning home; he indicated there was no one there who would be able to care for him. I wondered if he was afraid of leaving the security of the hospital. I felt my presence as an older professional woman (accompanying Caitlyn) created an audience for his anger, and it may have added to her sense of humiliation.

Irritability as a cover for vulnerability

Dennis, a black man in his early sixties with an African-Caribbean accent, had a strong-looking, compact body. He walked with two elbow crutches and was dressed in shorts and a t-shirt. Caitlyn asked how things were going for his discharge and he started to complain about his treatment. He said she wouldn't know about his difficulties as she had never been to his house to see what he needed. When she said she had called his wife to measure the height of the chairs, he seemed to become more agitated. He said that when his wife had previously been unwell, he had looked after her; he had to bathe her. He demonstrated how he had lifted her out of the bath (he cradled his arms as if lifting someone out of a bath) and asked: who would do that for him?

Caitlyn tried to reassure him, asking about a chair he could sit on in the lounge, but he became more agitated and said, 'What chair . . . what chair?', adding, 'Who will move my chair? Who will help me?' With this he wasn't looking at her but seemed to be appealing to me to understand that the help he had been given up to this point had not been of any use – he also seemed to be asking Caitlyn to 'do something'. It seemed that it didn't matter what Caitlyn suggested; it wasn't going to be good enough. He kept saying that she should have been to see his house for herself. I had an image of a small boy who didn't want to leave school – he had probably received a lot of praise from the staff for 'getting better', and didn't want to miss the special attention he got for his recovery.

Caitlyn was visibly shaken after this tirade and she went through to the nurses' office and began to cry. She said she didn't understand why he had been so upset and that she had done the same for him as she did with all the other patients who had had 'elective surgery', as if doubting her professional ability. When a nurse came in and saw she was crying, she said that Dennis had been 'like that' since he had heard he was being discharged. She said she didn't think he wanted to go home.

During the observation period I had a dream about my father, who had died 10 years earlier in a hospital. At the age of 65 he had gone for elective surgery on his femoral artery, and following the operation he had been allowed up to walk to the bathroom and he had died instantly from a heart attack, as a blood clot was dislodged and entered his heart. It had been a deeply shocking event for my family and I wasn't aware of thinking about it until I realised that, with each of the older men I saw in the hospital, I would look for my father. I imagined how he would have been very irritable with any request from a female therapist to demonstrate his skill in being 'independent' in his self-care.

The observation period brought several areas of enquiry that were explored in the later interviews (FANIs) with occupational therapists. Some of these themes were: the difficulty for young women in working with older male clients; witnessing physical frailty; and the fear clients expressed, overtly or covertly, about the 'power' occupational therapists had in deciding their future; that is, in their discharge planning. It had seemed to me that one way occupational therapists managed this complex emotional field was to focus on the physical capability of clients (walking, toileting, washing) and/or to offer equipment to assist clients in these tasks.

Not many of the occupational therapists seemed able to acknowledge the clients' emotional experience of the fear of being in hospital or the sense of humiliation and shame at needing the help offered. I considered that the emphasis on 'giving equipment', which was tantamount to prescribing it, could have been an unconscious social defence that occupational therapists used to protect themselves from the responsibility they carried. For example, the 'assessments' and clinical judgements therapists made could irrevocably alter where clients would live after leaving the hospital. I wondered if keeping the tasks at a functional level 'reinforced an unconscious denial of the horror of becoming old; i.e. the loss of one's bodily integrity (e.g. incontinence) and increasing physical dependence on others' (Nicholls, 2009, p. 176).

As mentioned above, following the death of my father in hospital many years earlier, I wasn't expecting to find it painful to observe the older men in the wards, but these associations helped me think about the anxiety of these clients in a hospital ward. In looking back through my notes from the observations, I was able to develop themes for further enquiry during the second part of the research, the free association narrative interviews (FANIs). These would sometimes include offering an interpretation of what I had seen or of what they had been saying.

Interviews, interpretation and ethical endeavours

In Hollway and Jefferson's (2000) description of developing and using the FANI, they explicitly state that the researcher must be careful *not* to make interpretations of what is said by the participant. In many ways their method allows for these interpretations to take place later: for example, when the written data are analysed and presented in research publications. I found, when listening to the first few recorded interviews I had undertaken, that the dialogues were littered with my interpretations. I would find that I offered suggestions (or interpretations) as to what the actions or words of the participant (or client) may have meant. Mostly I would do this as a form of a question: for example, when discussing a team leader's (Alison's) professed need to care for her clients and staff, I asked 'Do you think that occupational therapists are sometimes afraid of their own vulnerability?' This question led on to Alison's description of her childhood experiences of living with a depressed mother, whom she was required (emotionally and physically) to care for.

Within the FANI method of interviews, Hollway and Jefferson (2008, 2000) suggested that there was much to be gained from undertaking two interviews, using the intervening time (of a week) to listen to and reflect on the material from the first interview. These reflections may include identifying feeling tones, missed opportunities and possible resistances in, or between, the participant and researcher. In the book *Researching beneath the Surface* (Hoggett and Clarke, 2009), on psychosocial research methods, I attempted to justify my use of interpretations in using the FANI narrative method:

> There may be opportunities in the FANI which allow for the researcher to test a hypothesis (a selected fact or overvalued idea) that they have been considering within the research and with the participant. I found this particularly useful in the second interview where I could explore notions that had occurred to me during the first interview and while listening to the recording.
>
> (Nicholls, 2009, p. 181)

The following example is taken from an interview with Caitlyn. I had previously noticed that when she was telling me about a client she would give detailed case material using medical terminology. I had wondered if she used this language as a way of distancing herself from the client's injury, which may have been shocking to see or hard to imagine. When I had asked her if she ever felt disturbed or distressed when working with an elderly person or witnessing a traumatic injury, she replied that she 'doesn't think about it'. In the second interview (FANI) with Caitlyn, she described her experience of working with a younger man who had had a traumatic amputation (i.e. an unexpected amputation as a result of an accident).

Too close for comfort

Caitlyn: I have an amputee, a chap who has a lower limb amputation and he is about in his fifties. I think I find it harder to relate to him . . . than I do the elderly.

Lindsey: When you talk to him . . . do you ever find yourself getting in contact with his shock, his shame, his sense of bewilderment about the loss of a body part . . . [or] as you say 'you don't think about that'?

> **Caitlyn:** [laughs] Maybe . . . that is where I try to stop being an occupational therapist and start thinking more medical like, [laughs] . . . yeah and that's probably where being around the doctors in such an acute environment, you try to think about it just as a diagnosis . . . I know it sounds hard. Obviously when you are with the patient you are aware of how it affects them . . . but yeah . . . I do . . .

In the excerpt above, Caitlyn seems to being saying two things: that it is easier for her (emotionally) to treat the patient like a 'doctor' – that is, as a symptom or diagnosis – but that 'she is aware of how it affects him'. She says that it was harder for her to work with him than working with older patients. I wondered if the young patient was too close in age for her to maintain the distance she felt possible with frail, elderly clients. Perhaps his accident may have symbolically represented for her that she too was vulnerable, fallible and mortal.

The advantage of immersing myself in the culture of a group of occupational therapists was that I could form close relationships with the participants and this empathic involvement allowed me to risk some 'interpretations' (like the one I presented to Caitlyn above). Sometimes, by offering my thoughts and associations to the material, new thoughts and insights would emerge, and sometimes my interjections would be dismissed out of hand. 'I had thought that because the participant was not in an ongoing relationship with me, if my interpretations were clumsy and/or inaccurate they wouldn't be harmful . . . In my experience the interpretations I used assisted the interview more often than hindered it and what was not tolerated (i.e. thought about) by the participant was easily dismissed, often to my considerable chagrin!' (Nicholls, 2009, p. 181).

The use of interpretation to extend the narrative interview (through associations and reflections) is eloquently described by Hoggett *et al.*'s (2010) account of their biographical research into 'development workers'. They used the FANI and found, in a similar way to my experience, that it was the response of the participant that confirmed (or not) the usefulness of their interpretations.

> . . . when the epistemic alliance between interviewee and interviewer is working well, firm evidence of the value of an interpretation can be found from the ways in which interviewees respond. Here there is a precise parallel with psychoanalysis: a good interpretation produces new material, or it enables new connections to be made within what is already known . . . the extent that the 'truth value' of a formulation can be judged according to its capacity to generate new insights . . . we endeavour to illuminate our interviewees' unique, personal experiences of the social relations that form them and are formed by them.
>
> (Hoggett *et al.*, 2010, p. 183)

Beneath the surface

Researching the suggestions of unconscious motives in the participants (and researchers) requires methods that are able to reach beyond actions and dialogues that are seemingly within conscious control. Over the last few years, there have been examples of studies which employ the clinical psychoanalytic methods (e.g. dream analysis, free association, art or play) as research methods to gain an understanding of the hidden dynamics in individual choices, social groups and/or cultural events. Manley (2009) used social dreaming for a group of Bristol residents/participants to explore their understanding (i.e. associations and knowledge) of the history of slavery in Bristol. Burman (2010) has used art, the participants' and her own, to explore the function of containment in traumatised South African youth. Urwin (2007) has been part of a 3-year project (Hollway, 2007) that used the linked method of infant observation and free association narrative interviewing to understand the multiple changes in identity that first-time mothers experience in the multiethnic community of Tower Hamlets (London).

In my research project, I invited participants to share dreams they had about their work. The following dream, narrated by an experienced team leader, Diane, seemed to echo many of the themes that were part of the unconscious life (social defences) of an occupational therapy culture.

Dreaming the cat: ambivalence towards care work

In the dream she had hiked to the top of a steep mountain and as she was descending she saw something lying to the side of the path. She was with friends; she didn't recognise them but knew they were friends of hers. She went off the path and it was very steep and dangerous, and lying on the ground was a kitten that was also a baby. She picked this kitten/baby up and it had broken bones; she held it very still against herself and realised that if she moved it would die. She was wearing socks not shoes and it had started to rain. The path was very slippery and she tried to take off her socks without moving the bundle held against her chest. She walked down the mountain holding this kitten/baby. It was starting to get dark and she was worried that she would hurt this baby further.

Her friends didn't help her; they didn't seem to notice that she was struggling. When she got to the bottom of the mountain, she walked up to a building where there was a light on and a swing door to get in. As she stepped up on to the veranda to walk through the door, she missed the step and tripped, dropping the baby/kitten. As it fell to the ground, she realised that the fall would probably kill it and she felt terrible (grief-stricken) and relieved at the same time. She woke up as the baby/kitten fell and she remained feeling this mixture of emotions.

I said the dream seemed to be about her work; after all, the orthopaedic patients had broken bones. Diane said she hadn't made that connection. She asked me why I thought her friends hadn't helped her. I asked if in the dream she had asked them; she smiled and said no, she hadn't – it was like her not to ask for help.

Although this dream may have said much about Diane's personal internal world, it echoed some of the themes which had begun to emerge from the enquiry groups and individual interviews. As Lawrence (1998, 2003) in his work on 'social dreaming' has suggested, certain dreams can have a societal significance: that is, they represent a cultural concern or defence. In other words, if Diane's dream was a shared symbol of a common cultural defence amongst occupational therapists, what could it offer as a way of understanding the hidden (below the surface) aspects of working as an acute care occupational therapist? Could it have suggested that, while therapists offered help and support for their clients, they were unable to recognise this as a need inside themselves? Experiences of vulnerability were more easily located in the 'other' (clients and/or partners and friends), but the resulting dependence could be terrifying. Did occupational therapists, beneath the professional expression of care and concern, have strong paradoxical emotions of relief and grief when the client died or recovered?

Ethical endeavours

In the current climate of recognising the importance of service user involvement in developing research designs – 'nothing about me without me' (Department of Health, 2010, p. 3) – I have wondered how the ethics of consent and beneficence could be employed. Can psychoanalytic research be undertaken where the analysis and interpretation given to actions and/or narratives seem to take place without the participants' active acknowledgment or consent?

> The problem of whose 'voice' was being represented (and the ownership of information) was partially solved if the researcher shared their understanding of the analysis of the social defences, with the participants . . . [This may] . . . support the whole inquiry process by including insights of the participants to the hypotheses generated through the analysis. But is sharing of psychological 'insights' ethical'?
>
> (Nicholls, 2009, p. 183)

In addition to the issue of whose 'voice' is represented is the concern over the intimate nature of relationships established between researcher and participant by using in-depth interviews. Do these methods potentially 'harm' the participants? Huisman (2008) describes such an ethical dilemma in her description of developing relationships with a marginalised group (Bosnian Muslim refugee women) whose voices were seldom heard or represented in society. They viewed her as a 'friend', whereas she knew she would leave when the project was complete. She described her work with Mirsada, a lonely (isolated) woman, and her ethical conflict about what these research meetings had meant for Mirsada.

> On many occasions, we would get started on the interview, but then one thing would lead to another and we never seemed to get very far. Then, on one cold and dreary winter day, Mirsada offered to finish the interview. Two hours later, after she had shared some of her most private thoughts with me, she looked at me and asked, 'Does this mean that you are not going to come

visit me anymore?' . . . I feared that what I was doing ran counter to my
commitment to feminist ideals of equality, reciprocity, and improving the
lives of women.

(Huisman, 2008, p. 388)

Huisman (2008) does not believe there is one type of methodology that can solve these ethical dilemmas and concerns. She stated that ethics need to go beyond what is 'promised', through information sheets and letters of consent, to participants (or service users). Ethical consideration relies on the authentic commitment by the researcher to interrogate the purpose of the methods that they use to gather information. They need constantly to reflect on their personal or professional reasons for undertaking the study, and use supervision and reflexive activities (writing, dreams and associations) to remain available to the experience of the 'other': that is, the research participant and/or the culture of the organisation.

Kleinman (1988) and other recent social scientists (e.g. Clouston, 2003; Oritz, 2001) have identified that in the process of being researched, the participant can experience a positive therapeutic effect. They have suggested that the relationship and methods used in research that elicited narratives from clients of 'lived' experiences, given to a sensitive and emotionally responsive researcher, provided the participants with an opportunity to make sense of their losses and/or their lives. As Oritz (2001) stated, this positive outcome was unexpected in his research into the life world experiences of the wives (or partners) of professional athletes.

. . . the interview sessions seemed to provide several of the wives with
cathartic opportunities for self-revelation and introspective opportunities
for self-discovery, both of which may possibly contribute to a potential for
transformation in self and identity.

(Ortiz, 2001, p. 193)

The researcher's skill in finely attuned listening and responding, summarising themes or identifying underlying emotions, is the basic tenet of any ongoing therapeutic relationship. It is the substance of any long-term clinical work and perhaps by incorporating some of the psychoanalytic research methods (described above) an evidence-based practice may be closer to hand than many clinically focused therapists have realised. After all, Freud's original theories and methods grew from his desire to relieve the mental suffering in his patients.

Learning from the participant

This chapter has focused on the epistemological reasons for considering a psychoanalytic approach to research. It has suggested which methods can be used and offered examples of research where these methods have been used, but what about psychoanalytic research in occupational therapy? Peloquin (2005), in her Eleanor Clarke Slagle lecture to the American Association of Occupational Therapists, quoted Ora Ruggles, a therapist working with injured soldiers from the First World War: 'It is not enough to give a patient something to do with his hands [Ora Ruggles said.] You must reach for the heart as well as the hands. It's the heart that really does the healing' (Peloquin, 2005, p. 69).

In this final section I would like to draw the reader's attention to a selection of studies in occupational therapy that can help us understand the experience of the patient, carer and/or health professional. Through this work we are able to gain an emotional awareness of the person, their illness and its affect on relationships and their identity; in this process we learn something of ourselves and a shared humanity. As I have said to undergraduate students, we know we have learnt something, not only because we can recall it, but because we are changed by understanding it. There are many examples from occupational therapists who, in writing about their work with patients, evoke our moral imagination and expand our emotional awareness of the 'other'.

Kinsella (2006) wrote a powerful account of her work with a terminally ill, attractive young female patient, called 'Louise'. Kinsella explored her own unconscious reluctance to emotionally engage with the client, thereby protecting herself from the inevitable loss. It is an honest and deeply moving article that teaches us that being 'professional' can sometimes be used as a shield to keep the patient at an emotional distance. This can hurt the patient, but as Kinsella acknowledged, it can hurt the therapist too.

Using a different research medium, Salmon (2006) wrote a heart-rending autoethnographic description of her experience in caring for her demented mother. This very personal (reflexive) account conveys the painfulness of memory loss, the carer's anger related to past hurts that can become ever present, and the relief and guilt at handing the responsibility of the care work to institutional staff.

In her doctoral study of occupational therapists working in a spinal cord rehabilitation unit, Mattingly (1998) described how the occupational therapists were able to weave narratives of future possibilities within a client's current and (often) pessimistic view of their limitations. Clouston (2003) encourages OTs to use their knowledge of the client to record their narratives as a way of capturing, translating and transforming the experience. The research becomes an activity for the client through which they can (potentially) make sense of their illness experience.

Psychoanalytic thinking in research begins with considering the participant as having a complex, often conflicted inner life that is present in their conscious and unconscious communication. It is a way of thinking about human beings and their relationship with each other (and the researcher). This approach to understanding people brings new developments to existing ethnographic methodologies: observation, interviews and/or enquiry groups. It sometimes requires an intuitive leap of the imagination, as the researcher listens to what is being said with their head and heart. This detailed analysis of the everyday events in clinical practice can become the data used for research.

Cunningham and Gibertoni (Chapter 11) have used Interpretative Phenomenological Analysis (IPA) to interrogate the data they gathered from interviews with postgraduate occupational therapy students and clinical therapists. Most of the chapters in this book have detailed clinical examples of the long-term therapeutic work the authors have undertaken with clients. The accounts of their sensitive nuanced interventions demonstrate the significant change that is possible when time, attention and a place to experiment with activities is made available (see Gibertoni in Chapter 3; Cunningham in Chapter 4; Daniel in Chapter 5). As Cunningham and Gibertoni describe, their psychoanalytic theoretical/practice model (MOVI – see Chapter 7) developed from many years of clinical work, detailed group discussions and collaboration with analytic therapists. Their work is an exceptional illustration of how ongoing clinical work, through the use of theory, peer discussions and supervision, can develop into theoretical models for practice.

Conclusions

It is hoped that this chapter will encourage more clinical therapists and social science researchers to consider using some of the methods that have evolved through incorporating psychoanalytic theory into research methodology (e.g. the FANI). At the simplest level, it is a method for recording the experiences of clients and/or working with clients. This witnessing and transcribing of experience, the clients' and our own, *is* research. It can make the invisible, visible; it is a form of valid evidence and by capturing it (through the methods described above and publication), it can enrich the whole profession.

References

Bick, E. (1964) Notes on infant observation in psychoanalytic training. In A. Briggs (ed.), *Surviving Space* (pp. 37–54). London: Karnac, 2002.

Burman, H. (2010) Active witnessing: Lefika la Phodiso's response to the South African xenophobic crisis. *Journal of Psycho-Social Studies*, 4 (1), 6–31.

Clarke, S. (2003) *Social Theory, Psychoanalysis and Racism*. Basingstoke: Palgrave Macmillan.

Clarke, S. (2006) Theory and practice: Psychoanalytic sociology as psycho-social studies. *Sociology*, 40 (6), 1153–1169.

Clarke, S., and Hoggett, P. (2009) *Researching Beneath the Surface*. London: Karnac.

Department of Health (2010) *Equity and Excellence: Liberating the NHS*. London: The Stationery Office.

Clouston, T. (2003) Narrative methods: Talk, listening and representation, *British Journal of Occupational Therapy*, 66 (4), 136–142.

Finlay, L. (2002) 'Outing' the researcher: The provenance, process, and practice of reflexivity. *Qualitative Health Research*, 12 (4), 531–545.

Finlay, L. (1998) Reflexivity: an essential component for all research? *British Journal of Occupational Therapy*, 61 (10), 453–456.

Freud, S. (1919) *The Standard Edition of the Complete Psychological Works of Sigmund Freud*, Vol. XVII: *An Infantile Neurosis and Other Works*. London: Hogarth Press and the Institute of Psychoanalysis, 1975.

Gilbert, N. (2001) *Researching social life* (2nd edn). London: Sage.

Hammersley, M. (1992) *What is Wrong with Ethnography?* London: Routledge.

Hammersley, M., and Atkinson, P. (1995) *Ethnography* (2nd edn). London: Routledge.

Hinshelwood, R. D. (2002) Applying the observational method: Observing organisations. In A. Briggs (ed.), *Surviving Space* (pp. 157–171). London: Karnac.

Hoggett, P., and Clarke, S. (2009) *Researching beneath the Surface*. London: Karnac.

Hoggett, P., Beedell, P., Jimenez, L., Mayo, M., and Miller, C. (2010) Working psycho-socially and dialogically in research. *Psychoanalysis, Culture and Society*, 15 (2), 173–188.

Hoggett, P., Beedell, P., Jimenez, L., Mayo, M., and Miller, C. (2006) Identity, life history and commitment to welfare. *Journal of Social Policy*, 35 (4), 689–704.

Hollway, W. (2001) The psycho-social subject in 'evidence-based practice'. *Journal of Social Work Practice: Psychotherapeutic Approaches in Health, Welfare and the Community*, 15 (1), 9–22.

Hollway, W. (2007) Afterword. *Infant Observation*, 10 (3), 331–336.

Hollway, W., and Jefferson, T. (2000) *Doing Qualitative Research Differently*. London: Sage.

Hollway, W., and Jefferson, T. (2008) The free association narrative interview method. In L. M. Given (ed.), *The SAGE Encyclopaedia of Qualitative Research Methods* (pp. 296–315). Sevenoaks, CA: Sage.

Huisman, K. (2008) 'Does this mean you're not going to come visit me anymore?': An inquiry into an ethics of reciprocity and positionality in feminist ethnographic research. *Sociological Inquiry*, 78 (3), pp. 372–396.

Hunt, J. (1989) *Psychoanalytic Aspects of Fieldwork*. Sage University Paper Series on Qualitative Research Methods 18. Newbury Park, CA: Sage.

Kinsella, A. (2006) Poetic resistance: Juxtaposing personal and professional discursive constructions in a practice context. *Journal of the Canadian Association for Curriculum Studies*, 4 (1), pp. 35–49.

Kleinman, A. (1988) *The Illness Narratives*. New York: Basic Books.

Krog, A. (2009) My heart is on my tongue – the untranslated self in a translated world. In P. Bennett (ed.), *Cape Town 2007, Journeys, Encounters: Clinical, Communal, Cultural – Proceedings of the 17th International IAAP Congress for Analytical Psychology* (pp. 133–147). Einsiedeln: Daimon.

Kvale, S. (1999) The psychoanalytic interview as qualitative research. *Qualitative Inquiry*, 5 (1), 87–113.

Lawrence, W. G. (1998) *Social Dreaming @ Work*. London: Karnac.

Lawrence, W. G. (2003) Social dreaming as sustained thinking. *Human Relations*, 55 (5), 609–624.

Mackenzie, A., and Beecraft, S. (2004) The use of psychodynamic observation as a tool for learning and reflective practice when working with older adults. *British Journal of Occupational Therapy*, 67 (12), pp. 533–539.

Manley, J. (2009) When words are not enough. In S. Clarke and P. Hoggett (eds), *Researching beneath the Surface* (pp. 79–98). London: Karnac.

Mattingly, C. (1998) *Healing Dramas and Clinical Plots: The Narrative Structure of Experience*. Cambridge: Cambridge University Press.

Nicholls, L. (2009). Seeing ↔ believing, dreaming ↔ thinking: Mapping of methodological viewpoints. In P. Hoggett and S. Clarke (eds), *Researching beneath the Surface* (pp. 169–192). London: Karnac.

Nicholls, L. (2010) 'Putting it into words': A psychoanalytically orientated ethnographic study of hospital based clinical occupational therapy departments: in the UK and South Africa. Unpublished PhD thesis, University of the West of England, Bristol

Oakley, A. (2007) *Fracture: Adventures of a Broken Body*. Bristol: Policy Press.

Ortiz, S. M. (2001) How interviewing became therapy for wives of professional athletes: Learning from a serendipitous experience. *Qualitative Inquiry*, 7 (2), 192–220.

Peloquin, S. (2005) The 2005 Eleanor Clarke Slagle Lecture: Embracing our ethos, reclaiming our heart. *American Journal of Occupational Therapy*, 59 (6), 611–625.

Pillow, W. (2003) Confession, catharsis, or cure? Rethinking the uses of reflexivity as methodological power in qualitative research. *International Journal of Qualitative Studies in Education*, 16 (2), pp. 175–196.

Rustin, M. (1989) Observing infants: Reflections on methods. In L. Miller, M. Rustin and J. Shuttleworth (eds), *Closely Observed Infants* (pp. 52–75). London: Duckworth.

Salmon, N. (2006) The waiting place: A caregiver's narrative, *Australian Occupational Therapy Journal*, 53, 181–187.

Skogstad, W. (2004) Psychoanalytic observation – the mind as research instrument. *Organisational and Social Dynamics*, 4 (1), 67–87.

Urwin, C. (2007) Doing infant observation differently? Researching the formation of mothering identities in an inner London borough, *Infant Observation*, 10 (3), 239–251.

Young, D. (2006) Dennis Brown Essay Prize: How does group analysis work? *Group Analysis*, 39 (4), 477–493.

11 Understanding the Use of Emotional Content in Therapy Using Occupational Therapists' Narratives

Julie Cunningham Piergrossi and Carolina de Sena Gibertoni

The aim of this chapter is to examine closely the emotional content always present in therapy using the Vivaio model (MOVI), through the narratives of therapists who have worked with it for many years. (The model is described and discussed in Chapter 7.)

Introductory considerations

MOVI started out in a clinical situation and grew out of many years of working with emotionally disturbed children and adolescents. Our research (beginning 35 years ago) had a classical psychodynamic approach, starting with clinical experience, to which was added reflection, sharing, supervision and writing articles. These publications were always based on the application of theory (occupational, developmental and psychoanalytic) to a lived occupational therapy practice. In the beginning, the learning came from the children and young people who were in treatment, many of whom were seriously ill. They were the ones who helped us ask why the choosing and doing of things together was so effective in the healing process. We wondered how the emotions of the children and the therapists sometimes seemed to enhance and sometimes to hinder the therapeutic progress. The early writing focused on questions and we used theory to articulate our understanding of the unfolding process. Some of this work examined sensory experience and inner images (Gibertoni, 1991), the link between reality and the inner world (Cunningham Piergrossi, 1992), and activities and inner

Psychoanalytic Thinking in Occupational Therapy: Symbolic, Relational and Transformative, First Edition.
Lindsey Nicholls, Julie Cunningham Piergrossi, Carolina de Sena Gibertoni and Margaret A. Daniel.
© 2013 John Wiley & Sons, Ltd. Published 2013 by John Wiley & Sons, Ltd.

transformation (Cunningham Piergrossi and Gibertoni, 1995). Our own psycho-analytic training enlarged the field of study, self-reflection and application of psychoanalytic theory in our work as occupational therapists.

Our research was further elaborated through the training and supervision of other occupational therapists in the same approach, and this led to further learning from our students' questions, creativity, difficulties and discoveries. The model (MOVI) grew from this cycle of clinical observation, psychoanalytic theory, reflection, supervision, writing and training.

This chapter is based on the results from two studies which represent a further phase of learning. The studies use a qualitative research methodology to understand the complex world of doing, emotion and relationship in the occupational therapy process and the potential use of MOVI in facilitating this process. The results of the two studies will be discussed here using the narratives of 15 occupational therapists experienced in using the model. Both studies had a phenomenological orientation and utilised a semi-structured interview format.

Part 1: The lived experience of MOVI

In our first study (Cunningham and Gibertoni, 2006), we wanted to examine closely how our model was being applied by people who had completed the training and had been using it for a number of years in different kinds of setting. We chose just to let them talk about it for about 45 minutes to an hour, asking questions ourselves as they came naturally to mind during the conversation. In these conversations, both of us as interviewers were moved by the comments of our former students and found that they opened many opportunities for reflection.

The therapists

Vera was one of our first trainees and had been a physical therapist for several years before her rehabilitation hospital suggested taking our course in order to add occupational therapy to the hospital's treatment programme. She was interested but not sure she wanted to leave her solid physical therapy identity, and at the beginning of the course she worked part time as an occupational therapist (OT) and part time as a physical therapist (PT). At the end of our course she was ready to work full time in the new occupational therapy department in her hospital and began to train other therapists as well as describing the change that had come about in herself. 'MOVI opens the mind,' she explained. 'You see the person and not the pathology and this is a huge step because from then on you pay attention to the person, their choices and activities, which become much more than mere functions to be taught. To be able to consider the emotional aspects of my work, which are usually given little attention because they are feared by the health professionals, this helps me a lot.'

Giorgia was a nursery school teacher before taking the MOVI course because she wanted to be able to care better for children with special needs. In the course of time, besides changing the approach to the children in the classroom as a whole, she managed to create a special room in the school for working with disturbed children. 'Being sensitive and empathetic was not sufficient to work with children with special needs. The Vivaio course helped me to rethink the quality of the relationships between the children, the contents of the space and to see the behaviour of the children with new eyes.'

Lucia worked in a local paediatric neuro-psychiatric centre as a psychomotor therapist before taking the MOVI course. She had an excellent preparation in childhood neurological conditions but wanted to change and become an occupational therapist in order to use the relationship as a therapeutic tool. Lucia called the 3 years of the course 'a beautiful construction, a beautiful experience. Those were 3 years from which I came out changed.' She seems to be saying that the experience had helped her to build something new and solid, a construction both in the real world of her work and inside herself.

Chiara was a young physical therapist working with the elderly, when she came to the course looking for something she had not found in her former training; something that would help her to get really close to her patients who did not need physical therapy, but who needed something to help them go on living. She talked about the model as a basis for the treatment of all her patients, even those with whom she integrated other more functional models: 'It remains the foundation of my therapy because it takes into consideration the relationship between patient and therapist and this helps you to better understand how to go ahead in the therapy.'

Francesca worked in middle and high schools with young people with mental health and cognitive difficulties. She was able and creative in her work, but was looking for a framework, both practical and theoretical, to put her skills to better use. Upon finishing the course she opened her own private practice with children and adolescents. She described the discovery of a model which fitted into how she saw herself: 'I think that those who work with people and adopt a method do it because it corresponds to who they are, to their way of being; they feel it to be congenial. I liked the psychoanalytic approach, studying the cases in the details about what happened in each therapy session.'

MOVI as a change agent for the therapist

All of the therapists interviewed felt that the course had significantly contributed to changes in themselves which in turn became a basis for their way of working with patients. Vera put it this way: 'The Vivaio course helped me to change my attitude about the question of omnipotence. When you realise that you are not omnipotent, that you can't cure everything, that this realisation is not just verbalised but becomes a part of who you are, you realise that the little you can do can be good, can be a lot.'

Another change in themselves which the therapists noticed had to do with learning not to be judgemental. Of course, being judgemental is something most therapists try to avoid with their patients, but after their MOVI training the therapists interviewed seemed to understand better how to be non-judgemental in a more profound way and saw this as an important change in themselves. Lucia explained, 'Humility in the relationship means that I need to get to know you and that you need to get to know me but in a completely non-judgemental way.' Lucia's reference to humility in the relationship goes back to what Vera said about realising 'you are not omnipotent'.

The training lasted for 3 years and involved 4 hours of class work a week plus fieldwork experience. This long, steady learning experience, which included individual and group supervision, was the way we tried patiently to bring students from a rehabilitation background, where they had learned that there are always definable answers for resolving problems, to what Bion (1970) calls entering into therapy without memory and without desire. This is what we mean by being non-judgemental.

Chiara saw the same concept in her work with elderly persons: 'A relational approach means putting yourself on the same plane as the patients without judging them, being empathetic and trying to understand how I can be useful for them and what they are asking from the therapy.'

Working with the person and not with the pathology

Most of our students, and three of the therapists interviewed, came to the course after working in a medical setting where the emphasis of treatment was on the disease, the symptom and the medicine, and not on the person as a whole being. MOVI introduced them to a completely new way of working. In the words of Lucia: 'You try to reach a sense of harmony which can be experienced with words, with silence and with body language, but you don't go straight to the symptom.' Vera pointed out the difference between occupational therapy and other forms of medical help, and spoke from the patient's point of view: 'If you have an impairment and work on the impairment, you understand immediately why you are doing a certain exercise, but when there is an impairment and you work on something completely different, you might ask why you are doing it.' And saying this, Vera remembered the case of a young man, a former patient, who had complained to her that what she was doing was not important; all he needed was to walk. When he returned to visit her after leaving the hospital and getting a job he said, 'I wanted to tell you that I finally understand how useful occupational therapy was for me.'

Emotions about doing

The value of understanding and giving a voice to emotions during therapy was mentioned by all five of the therapists interviewed as central to their way of being with their patients.

Lucia talked about the objects that the children construct during therapy: 'The children's objects are an expression of feelings and truly a huge satisfaction and therefore give value to their feelings about themselves.'

In her work with the elderly, Chiara said that the Vivaio model helped them to live. 'Doing is very important; sometimes it even seems to stop time.' It seemed to us that Chiara was talking about working with the patients in a special moment of pause from life's troubles, in what Winnicott (1971) calls the intermediate space between one's inner world and outer reality where play and creativity reign supreme.

Francesca talked about doing as 'an expression of one's own inner desires and emotions and a way of finding solutions'. Giorgia described symbolic play as a powerful way to express emotion in children between 3 and 6 years of age. In her school, the parents of the children are invited to play as well. 'MOVI helped us to treat the relationship between parent and child, to think about the parents without judgeing them, to be open to their needs. Often, as a result, the parents seem to rediscover their own child because the life at school is different than that at home.'

The link between emotions and cognition when involved with activities was mentioned several times. Occupational therapists often work with children and adults with cognitive disabilities, and the objectives they establish need to be clear. Using MOVI, cognitive problems are not forgotten, but the relationship is the first priority. Francesca explains it this way: 'There are situations in which you realise that cognitive, learning aspects are important, but I never see these as my principal focus because they are inseparable from the emotional aspects. Children find many people who help them on a cognitive level, but almost never find someone who takes care of their subjectivity (i.e. their unique being).'

The therapist's recognition of emotions

The MOVI training is based on the premise that emotions, whether linked to the patient's outside life or about 'doing' in the relationship, must be recognised and given value by the therapist and never ignored. In many rehabilitation settings, emotions are considered difficult ingredients for the treatment and are only to be taken into consideration by psychologists, whereas MOVI teaches that emotions need to be recognised at the moment they appear.

Vera, who works in physical rehabilitation, claimed to have changed her attitude towards the patients: 'MOVI taught me to consider the emotional aspects of my work, which are usually given little attention because they are feared by the health worker. The patient wants to express himself and MOVI gives you the possibility of understanding both the verbal expression and the actions around what they choose or don't choose to do in the therapeutic setting.'

Choice of activity by the patient

Another basic concept of MOVI is personal choice on the part of the patient. The therapists agree that this is extremely important, though sometimes difficult, requiring the therapists to be very sure of themselves and their theoretical position.

According to Francesca: 'The element of choice is the thing that fascinates me the most, because since there isn't a path which is predictable, the therapy is more creative and permits the person more freedom.' Lucia adds a note of caution about the difficulties for the patients when confronted with the possibility of choosing: 'I always try to start from what the person wants to do but sometimes I suggest things to do when faced with someone unable to choose.'

Vera talks about the same kind of observation with her neurologically impaired patients, when the assessment period is finished and she tells them that now they have the possibility of choosing what they wish to do. 'This is almost always disorienting, because the idea is that to get better you have to do things that are dictated by someone who knows more than you do, who is part of the power structure. If this person tells you to do something in a certain way, you know it is good for you, but if you have to choose something for yourself, you cannot be so sure that it is right for you. On the other hand a person's autonomy, his or her roles in the family and in the community, are based on personal choice, and difficulties with this can be experimented in simple activities and faced and talked about with the therapist.' In her considerations Vera has struck on one of the very difficult aspects in medical settings of giving patients choices. She seems to be saying that when a person is hospitalised, he or she loses the habit of making significant choices for him or herself and slips into a dependent position in regard to the helping professionals. It seems to us to have to do with the importance of personal responsibility, a very complex psychoanalytic concept that in MOVI is often a point of arrival in therapy. Vera is telling us that patients need to take some responsibility for themselves and their choices while they are still in hospital.

Chiara speaks about the importance of the setting when offering the possibility of choosing: 'For older patients it's important to have a space where they can see the possibilities with their own eyes or see other persons who are involved in activities.'

Giorgia explains the changes occurring in many years of working with children and the value of observing and accepting the play choices of the children: 'The observation of the children's free play both singly and in small groups has helped us to truly discover them and to know them.'

Acceptance and closeness in the relationship

An important aspect of the intervention with MOVI has to do with a process of drawing slowly closer to the disturbed world of the patient, respecting his or her timing. This characteristic of the relationship with the patient is akin to being non-judgemental and expressing emotion, but different at the same time. Giorgia explained how it functions in the school setting: 'We observe the children and even when there are very difficult behaviours, such as aggressiveness towards objects or others, we give them time so that they feel accepted and not refused by the adult and their companions. The acceptance, the voice, the eye contact help the child to come closer and to feel safe, and slowly but surely a relationship is established.'

Francesca explained that the space and time of the therapy offers more control and is more controllable by the child than situations in everyday life. 'There are patients who take a long time to decide and they know they have a space and time for acceptance by a person who waits for their timing.'

The therapists are once again saying that their job is to try to come as close as possible to the child's world and not insist that he or she enter into theirs.

The influence of time

All of the therapists interviewed agreed that in MOVI having enough time is important. They see this as both a limit to and an advantage of the model. Vera described conflicting thoughts about time as a limit in the Vivaio model in a rehabilitation hospital: 'You need time to see changes in the patients because they represent things which mature with time; they are not the result of learning something, but personal inner changes. At a certain point, however, you realise that you do what you can, and with that, you don't worry about time any more.' Chiara is convinced that 'with experience you manage to use MOVI even with little time'.

Francesca saw the positive results of a long period of therapy: 'Being a model based on subjectivity it is by definition a long process and this could be considered a limit, especially in today's health scene. But this kind of therapy becomes a foundation, it lasts a long time, but it permits the patient to achieve results which last in time.' Francesca, in her work with disturbed children, has therapies that sometimes last for several years as she slowly works with both the children and their parents, accompanying them in a growth process that has been interrupted and helping them to understand behaviour and strong emotions, such as fear and anger, which can be very disruptive. Her point is well taken that once the therapy helps the child, step by difficult step, to take up the meaningful occupations in his or her life with new understanding, the results will last over time.

Reflections on the first study

The results of the first study raised a question in our minds about why a common theme in all the interviews concerned the training acquired during the 3 years of the MOVI course and the interviewees' emphasis on its incisive impact as a determining factor for their professional practice.

Much of the data seemed to indicate that learning about MOVI was a foundation, a source of enrichment, a chance for change, and had influenced their work in different clinical areas. In reflecting on this, we wondered if the training revealed itself to be the very essence of the model. It became clear that Lucia, Francesca, Giorgia, Vera and Chiara, during the course, had the chance to come in contact with their own emotions, to recognise them and to have less fear of them. This process of acquiring knowledge of one's own subjectivity came about through a series of experiences with doing and being which we have described elsewhere (see Chapter 12). These experiences enriched and changed, and constituted the beginning, the significant moment, the foundation from which each person could carry out the therapeutic roles requested of them.

We found that each of the therapists interviewed was able to join her own subjectivity to the subjectivity of her patients. This seemed to confirm the fact that, in the complex dynamics existing between patient, therapist and activity, it is the recognition of the emotional experience which constitutes the basic characteristic of the model and its clinical application. The five therapists emphasized the importance of this affective dimension, where the patient's 'doing' is an expression of the self (one's unique identity) and a dynamic element in the relationship with the therapist. The emotional and concrete elements of this therapy can be transformed into materials and products with form and meaning, which exist in their real form and have deep emotional resonance (Cunningham Piergrossi and Gibertoni, 1995). What the therapists are saying is that to recognise and get close to the emotions of the patient seems to become a kind of password for each and every therapeutic situation: for example, understanding the suffering of a loss, whatever it might be, might help the patient to retie the threads broken by the illness. In this way the rehabilitation process acquires a new dimension which is more meaningful, more human.

Part 2: The emotional significance of objects in therapy

The words from the poem 'Ode to things' by Pablo Neruda (1904–1973), in which he eloquently described his passionate love of so many treasured objects – buttons, wheels, garden shears (Neruda, 2003, p. 502) – seems to have been written for our second study (Cunningham Piergrossi and Gibertoni, 2010). The project was designed to investigate emotional investment in the environment, and in particular the significance of the objects, the physical touchable things, that are important to people during their occupational therapy experience. This was an aspect that had come out during the first study, and we were interested in knowing more in depth about what was happening in therapy sessions using MOVI in regard to objects.

The therapists

Ten experienced occupational therapists from diverse fields of the profession (five who worked with children, two who worked in adult neurological settings, one in geriatrics and two in adult mental health), who had previously been trained in MOVI, were asked to describe an object constructed or used in therapy which elicited a strong emotional investment from the patient. The participants were then asked to talk about the experience of working with the patient and their object, and to link the significance of the object to the therapeutic process.

All ten therapists interviewed said they had to think a while before deciding which object to describe, from the many that had been part of their work over the years. When describing the object and the person for whom it had been important, all ten were evidently still emotionally involved and seemed to ponder their stories carefully, wanting to make themselves understood by the researchers. Liliana talked about a papier-mâché egg; Elena, a purse; Francesca, a wooden ship; Giorgia, a wagon; Marta, colouring books, Lina, a plant; Pamela, a cardboard house; Agnese, a game of snakes and ladders with dice; Nadia, a personal diary; Susanna, a tape recorder. As with this eclectic group of 'things', each story was completely different but certain common characteristics began to emerge.

Turning point in the therapy

Almost all of the therapists talked about the objects they had chosen to describe as representing a turning point in the relationship and in the therapy itself.

One elderly patient, Maria, had begun to gather plants which had been abandoned around the geriatric institution where she was living and to bring them to the occupational therapy room to be replanted and cared for. 'From that moment Maria changed completely, her motivation towards the therapy increased immensely.'

Pamela described how, and only after a very long time, 7-year-old Matteo agreed to make a house out of a shoe box which happened to be on the table one day, and which became the object that permitted him to abandon the repetitive construction of clay snails and to grow through symbolic play. 'For the first months Matteo threw himself on the ground, hid in the cupboard or under the table and never responded to any question. The only thing he did was create little snails out of clay.'

Elena explains that a change came about in Anna after a long period of her needing to be cared for by the therapist, who mended her ruined clothes and gave her milk to drink. 'I proposed working together to knit a purse and I think this was the object that helped to click something into place in Anna. There was a change in her; the nurses were very surprised – she who only wore track suits now wanted to dress with a skirt and blouse.'

For 24 sessions, little 4-year-old Guido refused to acknowledge the presence of the therapist and passed quickly from one object to another without stopping or elaborating. With the introduction of the tape recorder he began to stop, to listen and eventually to initiate a form of symbolic play. 'At the twenty-fifth session I wanted to try to interrupt him in some way and turned on the tape recorder and called to him. We talked a bit together and he named his toy animals and then I played it back to him and he smiled and wanted to do it again.'

Liliana talked about Dario, a 14-year-old cognitively challenged boy in a wheelchair, who had progressive ataxic cerebral palsy. Before coming to occupational therapy he was extremely oppositional, repeating 'no, no, no' until he turned blue. The change came about very slowly, with his therapist permitting his 'no' and his not doing until they arrived at the construction of a papier-mâché Easter egg. 'From that moment on he couldn't wait to do other things, and he loves making and doing. I don't know how to describe it. He went from not wanting to do anything to hurrying to be able to do something.'

Francesca described a very long period of therapy with a regressed and primitive 7-year-old, Giuseppino, who expressed confused and fragmented feelings of loss in his play, before building a wooden ship which led to more mature play. 'I could feel his sense of loss and the summer holidays were approaching, and I was sorry because I knew that this separation would be difficult for him, so I suggested building a ship that he could take with him and he accepted.'

Marta described a situation which seems to be the opposite of the other therapists' experiences with the objects, in the sense that it was in letting go of an object, the colouring books that he repetitively filled, that 17-year-old Edoardo began to change and to grow. The therapist came to realise the reason these books had been so important for him: 'I was asking myself, what are we doing here? And now he gives me the answer, saying that the colouring relaxed him, freed his brain.' And she finished her tale by saying, 'It was very adult of him to allow himself to be so little.'

It was interesting for us to reflect on these kinds of magical moments in therapy, when things seem to take a change for the better without our always realising why.

In the cases described above, the therapists interviewed told how the presence of the object and the interaction between therapist, patient and object had given them a chance to focus on that moment of change in the patients themselves because it had been represented by change with the object. There was an inner change as well as a tangible visible change with a significant object. And we were reminded once again of the work of psychoanalyst Harold Searles (1960) on the unconscious significance of the nonhuman environment, including its objects; Searles described so beautifully how the emotional investment in nonhuman objects is tightly linked to human relationships.

> *The human being is engaged, throughout his life span, in an unceasing struggle to differentiate himself increasingly fully, not only from his human, but also from this nonhuman environment, while developing, in proportion as he succeeds in these differentiations, an increasingly meaningful related-ness with the latter environment as well as with his fellow human beings.*
> (Searles, 1960, p. 30)

Another consideration has to do with time and waiting – this is present in all of these examples and is often a dramatic aspect of the beginning of therapy. All of the therapists – some serenely, some with frustration – stayed with their patients, respecting their time needs, and had the impression that only in that way were they finally able to reach these very disturbed people, both old and young.

Emotional expression

Emotions were expressed around all of the objects described, but in some cases it was the object itself which helped either to unleash repressed emotion or to contain uncontrolled emotion.

Nadia described a patient who was extremely angry and oppositional, whose object helped her to control emotions which were causing problems for her with fellow patients and personnel on the ward. Paola was a 40-year-old woman who, after a car accident, had very limited verbal communication possibilities but no cognitive damage, and who was sent to occupational therapy to try to find some way of forming a relationship with her, to understand her 'difficult' behaviour. Paola, helped by the therapist, began to write her personal diary on the computer in spite of her severe motor difficulties, and her 'impossible' behaviour disappeared. 'This woman's crises of irritability, aggressiveness and crying were not understood by the persons who had contact with her on the ward and she was labelled as the classical difficult patient.'

Another therapist, Agnese, on the other hand, talked about an object that helped a very emotionally blocked patient to express repressed emotion. She described the board game of snakes and ladders, played with a 56-year-old man in a mental health day programme who was almost catatonic and used very few spoken words. She described the fear she could feel circulating in the room and the fear she felt herself; she even left open the door of the therapy room when he was there. 'At the beginning the game was the only way of expressing emotions, especially fear. We threw the dice and then I would put words to the emotions according to where the game would send us.' She described talking about fear that the dice would send her back to square one, about the feeling of triumph when she was ahead or frustration when he managed to shake a high number on the dice, and how he started expressing the same kinds of emotion.

When Pamela told the story of Matteo and his little cardboard house, she described how his violent father had terrorised both his mother and himself before being sent to prison. 'We came to the point of constructing a safe house and therefore to create a new story, a house that could be safe and with which he could start to put words to his emotions.'

Emotions of the therapist

It was very clear in the study how the emotional content invested in the object and its significance to the therapeutic relationship was felt by the therapists as well as by the patients. Sometimes the therapists were touched by aspects of their patients' behaviour that came as a surprise to them.

'I was very moved by their way of interacting during the preparation, and the impatience of one which was understood by the other.' These words from Giorgia, the only therapist interviewed who worked with a group, described two young boys who were constructing a wooden wagon. She was referring to the capacity of the young boy to have empathy for his companion, thanks to the wagon they were constructing together.

Nadia talked about her feelings connected to her very disabled patient's personal diary and how touched she was by how Paola began to communicate. 'I like to reread her diary; I look at the pictures and I feel like I can see Paola, and with strong emotion because when a woman cries as she writes about what has happened to her . . .'

Marta is the therapist who described her experience of the colouring books with Edoardo. She said she had grown almost to hate the object because she seemed unable to find any way to interrupt it. She only realised its importance a long time later. 'I was completely astonished when one day he abandoned the colouring books and started in on symbolic play. While playing he talked a lot about his problems, about not being like the others.' Edoardo was an adolescent with autism who needed the repetitive, autistic object of colouring books and a therapist ready to accept it before letting himself move on.

Symbolic meaning

The therapists interviewed seemed very aware of the symbolic content of their patients' communications with 'things', and transmitted their understanding in such a natural way that there seemed to be almost another dimension to their communication which went beyond words and was comprehended by both partners in the relationship. A good example of this is symbolic play, the essence of symbolic communication, which is so necessary in children's development.

Francesca told about 7-year-old Giuseppino who had been neglected and then abandoned by his mother, who ran off to San Marino (a tiny country inside Italy's borders). He had never talked about his mother and even in therapy never mentioned her, but now she was very present in a flag he placed on his wooden ship. 'He proposed to string a wire and to attach flags. He cut out the American flag and the Japanese flag and then asked me how the San Marino flag was made and we added that one as well.'

Matteo was another child who used his object for symbolic play, and as we listened to Pamela, his therapist, describe it, we could picture Matteo with his fears and his great need to control. 'He begins to construct the house with the shoe box, to cut out the windows, the doors, and slowly but surely this house takes form and becomes a house that needs emergency exits, burglar alarms and doors with padlocks, but they are never enough . . .' She explained how, further along in the therapy, in the symbolic play that was part of using the house she was nominated to be the guard. 'I had to control that there weren't holes in the floor and call to have things repaired that he had destroyed and I would say, "No, look, I had everything repaired well, it's indestructible." Sometimes he would accept and other times he would say, "It can't be indestructible if a meteorite or an earthquake arrives."'

Control is an important part of symbolic play; the children are the ones who control their lives while playing with a miniature world. They can also control adults – one thing they cannot do in the real world. Matteo in his play could control his therapist; sometimes he would accept her interventions and at other times he would let her know that he didn't consider her so strong, because an earthquake could always happen. She played with him and accepted his ambivalent feelings, but in a way that was fun and that included the play of both the child and the therapist. Winnicott (1971) considers the play areas of both members of the relationship to be fundamental in therapy and describes this as an overlapping of the play of the patient with that of the therapist.

Adults also communicate symbolically with their objects, sometimes telling more without words than they can express with a long verbal discourse. This is what Lina described in her story about the plant saved by her patient, Anna. 'I understood that what she was trying to tell me was that the little plant was she herself who was suffering for having been uprooted, torn from her house, her objects, from every-thing that was dearest to her, and that in that situation, if nothing were done, it would be the end.'

Competency feelings

So far our attention has been on the emotions, the symbols, the inner significance of objects, but objects also have a real value that can lead to the concrete realisation of abilities and a sense of competence that then increases the motivation for doing and being (White, 1959).

When Giorgia talks about her work with the two young boys who were constructing a wagon, she expresses a sense of wonder at how the growing competency of both contributed to a product that even she was surprised to see emerging. 'It was an experience that certainly called upon their fine motor skills, but also their creativity in decorating and painting it, and there was this great spirit of cooperation between them, each with different competencies.'

Agnese talked about how learning to count and to remember, and to dominate his fear of her in the game of snakes and ladders, helped her catatonic patient Signor Rossi to move towards competency experiences. By being able to express emotions in the game, he was able to be more flexible and allow himself to learn and try new experiences. 'Signor Rossi started coming on the bus by himself and a lot of other things as well.'

Elena underlined how important it was for her regressed patient Anna to 'be able', to let herself try. She seemed to have lost the natural tendency of human beings to interact with the world of things around her (White, 1959). She needed the relationship with the therapist to have the courage to see herself as someone who could do it. 'When I started with Anna she refused to do anything; she said she didn't know how to do anything. She said, "It's not worth the effort, I can't try", and even at the beginning with the purse she refused the cloth, the leather, everything I proposed.'

Describing the changes in 7-year-old Giuseppino, the therapist talked about the construction of the wooden ship and all of its meanings: 'He used the rasp and asked me, "Is this how cabinet workers do it?" He was trying out a role as a grown-up and invested a lot in the entire process of the construction.'

Reflections on the second study

Each of the objects described by the ten therapists tells a story, a story of a three-way relationship between therapist, patient and object. This three-way communication and its pivotal moment led the way to change. The stories are very different, but they all recount the intertwining of thoughts, emotions and choices that developed over time.

We were struck by the apparent simplicity of all of the objects; they were neither dramatically different from the many used or created in the therapy room, nor particularly creative, but they were objects which impacted on the relationship and on the outcome of the therapy in a very meaningful way. The therapists were not interested in an attractive or 'finished' product, but described a kind of magic and surprise when the idea for an object or the change in the object seemed to appear almost from nowhere. We realised that the choice of the significant object or its use was never casual. Using a psychoanalytic framework, we can say that the inner world of the therapist had come in contact with that of the patient, and this allowed something to happen between the two of them. This happening occurred in the here and now of the therapy situation, where every relationship is unique and where each new moment can be a creation (Winnicott, 1971). This communication took place at a symbolic (unconscious) level, helped by the presence of the real object, and at a physical (conscious) level represented by the competency experiences that many of the patients described.

Each of the ten stories could have been a paper in itself, but laying them out side by side gave us the chance to think about how change comes about in occupational therapy using a relational model, MOVI, which focuses on the interaction between therapist, patient and object that is always part of 'doing'.

Returning to the poem 'Ode to things', Neruda (2003) seems to understand what happens in occupational therapy, to understand that the objects, constructed or used as the therapies described, came alive for both the patient and the therapist, and he or she with them. He writes about how his favourite objects were full of life, how they 'befriended' his existence (Neruda, 2003, p. 504).

Part 3: Closing reflections on what we learned from listening to therapists' narratives

Emotion, as agent of change in the therapist as well as in the patient, seems to be the simple message and challenge of the two qualitative studies of MOVI – beautiful, feared, cherished, unmeasurable emotion. What the studies seemed to be saying was that emotions were necessary for inner growth and learning, both in the therapists' own training and in their work with their patients. In all of the examples described by the therapists, emotions seemed to start off the growth process, and they could exist only in a relationship. As Daniel Siegel (1999) stated: 'When interpersonal communication is "fully engaged" – when the joining of minds is in full force – there is an overwhelming sense of immediacy, clarity and authenticity. It is in these heightened moments of engagement, these dyadic states of resonance, that one can appreciate the power of relationships to nurture and to heal the mind' (p. 337).

The therapists' stories confirmed one of the basic tenets of MOVI when they spoke to the subjectivity and uniqueness of each and every therapy session. The very nature of a model with a psychoanalytic theory base is contradictory to predicting results, because it is built on the subjectivity of the person in therapy. No one knows how a therapeutic journey based on subjectivity will proceed or where it will lead, and the fact of not knowing is what gives it its strength as a therapeutic tool. It is not the therapist who knows what is best to do, think or feel, but it is the therapist who accompanies the patient in his or her search for meaning and helps the patients to have faith in themselves. Psychoanalytic research is not about numerical results, because it is impossible to define and quantify inner emotions or relational aspects of life or subconscious phenomena (see Chapter 10 on psychoanalytic thinking in research).

Another concept underlined by the therapists in their narratives, a concept we had more or less taken for granted, but which now seems somehow even more important, has to do with patience and waiting. This is a simple concept but is not usually contemplated in occupational therapy models. With a psychoanalytic theory model, it is essential to be able to wait, to respect the patient's time, to 'be with'.

One of the limits of MOVI is the time that can be required to be effective with patients who find it hard to trust others. In today's public health sector, which puts pressure on its professionals to produce results in the shortest time possible, there seems to be little space for this long-term therapy work. So looking at the results of the qualitative research presented here, we can underline the fact that the therapists who have been trained in the use of MOVI are prepared to use a defined setting that offers choice and have also acquired a different way of looking at their work and at the person with whom they are working. These results may be applicable in different kinds of setting (e.g. home care, community work, families, groups of elderly, etc.) and using different time frames (consultations, short-term therapy, etc.).

We discovered that the women interviewed who had studied MOVI spoke of changes in themselves as therapists which led to new creative ways of being with patients. We do not know if we are talking about a conceptual practice model or about a therapeutic philosophy, perhaps both. Our future research will aim at addressing this question; at the moment it seems that we are talking about two levels of MOVI, one which aims at a particular setting with a psychotherapeutic orientation and one which aims at increasing psychoanalytic thinking in the profession as a whole, whatever the setting.

Conclusions

What then do we mean by psychoanalytic thinking, and how is it different from what we read about spirituality, often mentioned in other occupational therapy models? The difference (as we see it) is in the use of the relationship as an agent of change, which requires training, supervision and a particular interest in the human being's inner world. All of this requires time, but if it is of benefit to the patient, why not? Many occupational therapists who chose this line of thought, switched to a career as psychotherapists, leaving behind the activity (i.e. 'doing with') which was the essence of their occupational therapy profession. Many have acquired higher degrees in psychology and psychotherapy, but very few of these people have returned with their new skills to occupational therapy. Perhaps a higher degree in occupational therapy with a psychoanalytic orientation could be the answer. A whole new line of research could be born which would add a dimension to the profession which has always been there, but risks being ignored or neglected by more positivist, measurable ways of interacting with patients.

References

Bion, W. (1970) *Attention and Interpretation*. London: Tavistock.

Cunningham Piergrossi, J. (1992) Il reale. *Il Ruolo Terapeutico (rubrica Vivaio)*, 59, 50–52.

Cunningham Piergrossi, J., and de Sena Gibertoni, C. (1995) The importance of inner transformation in the activity process. *Occupational Therapy International*, 2 (1), 36–47.

Cunningham Piergrossi, J., and de Sena Gibertoni, C. (2006) The Vivaio model of occupation in the therapeutic relationship. Paper presented at the World Congress of Occupational Therapy, Sydney.

Cunningham Piergrossi, J., and de Sena Gibertoni, C. (2010) Emotional investment in the environment: Psychoanalytic research in occupational therapy. Paper presented at the World Congress of the World Federation of Occupational Therapists, Santiago, Chile, May.

de Sena Gibertoni, C. (1991) Sensi e immagini interne. *Il Ruolo Terapeutico (rubrica Vivaio)*, 58, 37–39.

Neruda, P. (2003) *The Poetry of Pablo Neruda*. New York: Farrar, Straus & Giroux.

Searles, H. (1960) *The Nonhuman Environment in Normal Development and in Schizophrenia*. New York: International Universities Press.

Siegel, D. (1999) *The Developing Mind: Toward a Neurobiology of Interpersonal Experience*. New York: Guildford Press.

White, R. W. (1959) Motivation reconsidered: The concept of competence. *Psychological Review*, 66, 297–333.

Winnicott, D. W. (1971) *Playing and Reality*. New York: Basic Books.

12 Training Experiences to Develop Psychoanalytic Thinking

Carolina de Sena Gibertoni

Introduction

This chapter looks at how the thinking and practice of working with emotions have been included in the Occupational Therapy curriculum at the University of Milan and in a private Master's programme. Recognition of feelings and emotions in our professional practice is central to our understanding of the client's communication and the complexity of coping with the three-way dynamic between patient, therapist and activity, a dynamic that can arouse and influence the choices we make in practice.

The Vivaio model, MOVI, discussed at length in Chapter 7, features specific learning experiences that aim to bring students closer to understanding and managing their affective states. Of these learning experiences, two will be described which are particularly significant. The first is a group experience using analytical psychodrama for students in the Occupational Therapy degree programme at the University of Milan, Italy. One of the aims of this teaching method is to uncover feeling states, reliving them by telling their story and playing out a scenic representation of personal interactions with patients, involving situations and feelings that may reflect a stalemate, a sense of overwhelming loss, or impotence.

The second learning experience is the mother–infant observation which is used with graduate occupational therapy students who are participating in the MOVI Master's course in Psychoanalysis and Occupational Therapy. One of the aims of this experience is to observe the birth of a relationship between mother and child and to study these observations in small seminar groups in which everybody contributes with comments on the material presented by each group member. In this way the participants become truly capable of observing and learning from real-life experiences. This chapter will describe the theory and process of each learning

Psychoanalytic Thinking in Occupational Therapy: Symbolic, Relational and Transformative, First Edition.
Lindsey Nicholls, Julie Cunningham Piergrossi, Carolina de Sena Gibertoni and Margaret A. Daniel.
© 2013 John Wiley & Sons, Ltd. Published 2013 by John Wiley & Sons, Ltd.

event, beginning with the use of psychodrama in undergraduate occupational therapy (OT) education.

Using analytical psychodrama for teaching

What is psychodrama?

In the famous painting, *Clinical Lesson of Doctor Charcot*, by Pierre-André Brouillet (1887), the scene depicted is of a patient with hysteria acting out the symptoms of her illness while the medics carefully observe and share the experience. On the one side, we can see the assistants; on the other, between Charcot and Babinsky, the patient known as the 'Queen of hysterics'. It is a painting that brings to light something that anticipates the birth of analytical psychodrama. This therapeutic technique was introduced by the Romanian psychiatrist Jacob Moreno (1889–1974), who lived in Vienna at the same time that Freud was seeking to understand the causes of hysteria in order to modify and improve the therapeutic approach. In 1920s Vienna, both Freud and Moreno created a link between psychoanalysis and theatricality, although with vast differences. Moreno believed in a scenic and visual therapy, a real theatrical performance, with an audience. The young actress Barbare, for example, who was considered to be the first psychodramatic patient, usually portrayed angelic roles, while in real life she behaved in a hysterical manner. When Moreno induced her to act out the part of a hysterical patient in front of an audience, Barbare improved greatly (Marineau, 1989).

Freud let his patients move, gesticulate and express opinions out loud, but in an enclosed space, not visible to strangers: the famous Anna O., for example, another psychodramatic prototype, staged her theatrics in private, in the absence of an audience (Breuer and Freud, 1892–1895; Freud, 1909). Although using very different approaches, both Moreno and Freud studied the link between hysterical gestures and hidden psychic movements, and investigated the relationship between psychoanalysis and dramatisation.

Ferenczi, in 1919, also introduced a technique by which he urged patients to stage real dramatisations, considering them to be tools to access the oldest psychic formations of the personality of the patient in question (Ferenczi, 1921).

It is as if the psychodrama created by Moreno had drawn in and integrated with other authors in the search for a relationship between psychopathology and scenic representation. Studies and research have developed throughout the last century by post-Freudian and Freudian authors on the subject of psychoanalysis, the subject of the connection between acting and psychoanalysis, and the subject of the study of group therapy (Anzieu, 1956; Kaes, 1972; Lemoine and Lemoine, 1973; Lebovici, 1974; Miglietta, 1998).

This confluence of ideas has been captured in the extraordinary works of D. W. Winnicott (1896–1971), who, with ingenuity and wisdom, introduced us to the concepts of play and of creativity, and of their relationship to psychotherapy (1971). He stated: 'psychotherapy takes place in the overlap of two areas of playing, that of the patient and that of the therapist . . . If the patient cannot play, then something needs to be done to enable the patient to become able to play, after which psychotherapy may begin' (Winnicott, 1971, p. 72). He went on to explain that 'in a tantalizing way many individuals have experienced just enough of creative living to recognize that for most of their time they are living uncreatively, as if caught up in the creativity of someone else, or of a machine' (p. 87).

Similarly, Melanie Klein (1882–1960), through the development of the mechanisms of projective and introjective identification and the introduction of child analysis, began using both play and dramatisation with children, thereby developing the theme of personifications and the invention of characters who followed an improvised script, subject to changes related to identifications with people and situations.

In 1929 Klein wrote:

> I also drew attention to one principal mechanism in games in which different 'characters' are invented and allotted by the child. My object in the present paper is to discuss this mechanism in more detail and also to illustrate by a number of examples of different types of illness the relation between the 'characters' or personifications introduced by children into these games and the element of wish-fulfilment.
>
> (Klein, 1929, p. 199)

After the insights of Winnicott and the personifications of symbolic play from Klein's individual therapies, many steps via numerous different theories were taken surrounding the meaning of play. They were joined together with Bion's group theory (Bion, 1961, 1962) and the concepts of container-contained (Bion, 1962) and reverie (Bion, 1962) elements that, in the group dynamics of psychodrama, facilitate the creation of an emotional–relational field, permitting the transformations of affective and mnemonic events and activating new connections between levels of reality and levels of thinking.

Today, analytical psychodrama is a valid tool in and for group analysis. Participants attend the sessions in a fixed space and time, and the meetings have a duration of 60–75 minutes. The group sits in a circle and the conductor or conductors accompany the free associations (Freud, 1911) of the participants with fluctuating attention (Freud, 1912), and carefully promote the dramatic play element which characterises this technique. The scene acted out in the course of the group session may include an exchange of actors, and it is here that numerous insights emerge and learning can occur. The session is not open to the public or to external observers: it is a closed group. At the end of the session, the conductor adds his or her understanding of what happened in this action method.

How MOVI uses analytical psychodrama

MOVI incorporates the methodology of analytical psychodrama [1] as an educational tool to bring occupational therapy students closer to an understanding of underlying

---

[1] Analytical psychodrama began to be used in Italy in the late 1970s. The Italian Society of Analytic Psychodrama began in 1981, but the founding group (Miglietta, Curi Novelli, Croce, Mele, and others) had been active since 1968 with the introduction of analytic psychodrama by the Lemoines, founding members of the Société d'Etude du Psychodrame Thérapeutique of Paris.

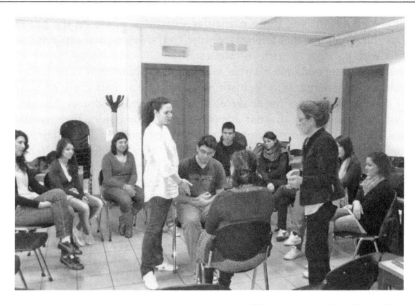

Figure 12.1 Psychodrama session for students at the "Università degli Studi" of Milan, Italy.

affective states in clinical situations arising from their fieldwork placements, which they present to their class group.

There are full descriptions of the theory and process of psychodrama in many textbooks (e.g. Kaes, 1972; Miglietta and Pani, 2006). For the purposes of this chapter, common psychodrama terms are used: for example, the therapist is called 'the conductor' and the student presenting their drama is called 'the protagonist'.

'There are no lights, no scenery, only a scene representing the "human element"' (Brook, 1995, p. 11). Without scenery, lights or a stage, but within a private space, the students act out scenes of human encounters with the first patients they have met on their paths to becoming occupational therapists. The meetings are difficult; the students talk about patients with severe brain damage, young patients without the use of arms or legs, stroke patients, schizophrenics, neurological problems, Alzheimer patients, children, adults, older people, a population of suffering never before encountered in their young lives. They tell and recreate, through scenic representation, the strong emotional impact that some episodes have had on them.

The experience which unites the group of students is not an analysis of the personal unconscious dynamics put into play by the participants, and it is not a form of clinical supervision by an experienced therapist from that area. It is a tool that enables an analytical way of working: a defined setting, respecting space and time, based on the telling of what happens during fieldwork placements with an eventual scenic representation and a conductor capable of 'reverie' (i.e. thinking about the experience), who is attentive to emotional experiences and the group dynamics that the experience brings to life.

The theoretical frame refers mostly to the concepts of projective identification and the thoughts found in Bion's seminal work, *Learning from Experience* (1962). Students are encouraged to concentrate on their fieldwork experiences and to try to recall moments of impasse, those particular situations where, in the presence of unmanageable emotions, they felt lost, confused or powerless and experienced a loss of contact with patients or with colleagues.

Within the setting, seated in a circle, students talk about their experiences, their relationship with patients, with the institution, with the activity itself, and how they felt. The conductor assumes the dual role of observer and conductor. She sits in the circle, listens, takes note of what happens and accompanies the narratives. If necessary, she invites participation in the play by directing the acting of role inversion, where the protagonist takes the part of other people in the drama (after that of the patient, so the protagonist can feel what the patient feels). The conductor gathers the experiences of the leading players and the experiences that each participant evoked in relation to their work situation.

The conductor also notes the differences between narration of the event and what occurred in the acting of it, including the mental states that emerged within the whole group via the interpersonal dynamics. The following example gives an idea of how the method is used to extend the students' emotional learning.

Role reversal: generating resonance and reflection

Simone speaks of a schizophrenic patient (Michele, aged 27) who had been assigned to him and who would refuse to do anything. He would sit inert on the couch, get up only to smoke or eat, and reject any suggestions made to him. Simone feels useless and powerless. One morning, finally, he manages to get him into the occupational therapy room and immediately suggests the idea of making a clay ashtray where he can put his cigarette ash. As Simone is handing him the block of clay, Michele grabs hold of it and throws it into his face. Surprised and with an aching face, Simone gets angry and scolds him severely, while Michele bursts into laughter.

Simone's story animates the group with comments and evokes memories of work experiences focused on the aggressiveness of patients and the feeling of powerlessness in trainees. The conductor invites Simone to enact the scene of the block of clay thrown into his face. After much uncertainty Sara is chosen to represent the patient, who is described as being tall, very thin and with a mass of long and ruffled hair. Sara is small and thin, but with a shock of red hair.

The play is very intense and highlights Simone's marked insistence that Michele should make the ashtray and the exasperating invitation at least to touch the clay. In the face of pressure from the trainee therapist, the student acting as Sara (in the role of Michele) feels impatient to the point that she raises her right arm in the act of throwing the clay at Simone. Simone gets angry and Sara bursts into a loud laugh. When the conductor suggests a total role reversal, where Simone becomes the patient and takes the role of Michele, he moves incessantly, plugs his ears with both hands and seizes the tail of his shirt as if he were about to rip it off, until with violence, in the act of throwing the clay at Sara (who is now acting the part of Simone the trainee), he almost delivers a punch in her face. But Sara does not become angry and Simone, who is stunned, does not laugh.

Pursuing the group discussion which follows each drama, Simone communicates that he was deeply affected – the change of role had made him appreciate that anger can lead to pressure like the kind he had imposed on the patient. Sara also agrees with Simone's comment and adds that she was very glad to have been chosen to represent Michele and that she had greatly enjoyed being able to retaliate and laugh while looking on at the anger her gesture had caused.

The group weaves its way through several comments, evoking various situations through multiple projections and identifications, with patients and with trainees, sometimes full of anguish. What comes to the surface is their feeling of uncertainty, which generates anxiety in relation to interacting and suggesting materials or activities, a 'doing' at all costs, an anxiety that can hamper the ability to listen and wait, often resulting in negative emotional states in their clients.

At the end of the session the conductor gives a summary of what happened and underlines the differences between Simone's story, which concealed his pressing insistence, and the play which instead brought it all out. This was expressed by Simone's body language when he acted the patient, restless and very irritated. The conductor also highlights the function of reverie by the group, whose evocative activities served as a containment, allowing the expression of deep emotional ambivalence, and a form for working through these feelings. The scene played by Simone and Sara conveyed different emotional states, including anxiety, aggression, retaliation, helplessness and distress, all recognised as belonging to the entire group, which reclaimed them and transformed them into emotions that can be used in any therapeutic process.

As we have just seen, in playing out the scenic representation of a personal interaction in a certain situation, the inversion (exchanging) of roles usually generates an increase in intensity and involvement in the protagonist and auxiliary egos. In addition, the entire group, in observing, moves with transferences from one character to another, remaining present in the moment of each scene that is under way. After playing the protagonist, the actors speak, evoke, and comment together with the other participants, who express their thoughts on what occurred: their identifications, resonances and general reactions. The conductor, during the whole of the session, will be attentive to how much the group is able to have a container function, which would allow the transformation of projective and introjective identifications in all of the participants.

The method used in discussing fieldwork follows the use in analytical psycho-drama of a formal structure and its rules: for example, the participants are seated in a circle, are free to speak and expect respectful listening; a fixed time and space is used; and the roles are identified by the protagonist. But in our case it is a group based on clinical work experience and not a self-insight therapeutic group. This possibility of bringing to the group situations related to the fieldwork experience, which includes relationships with patients, with the activities, the institution, colleagues, other professional figures in different institutions, while excluding any reference to personal events, allows reflective clinical learning.

The emergence of a reflective group

A group of 22 third-year occupational therapy students met for a period of 9 weeks to use this method of group sessions. In the beginning, the students appeared suspicious. They found themselves in a classroom structure different from the usual one: sitting in a circle, not at a table watching a lesson in front of them. In this group learning, they were close together; they could see each other, in the presence of a silent conductor who watched them and waited for them to speak. But they seemed almost inhibited, as if they dared not speak, and intimidated by the silence, they attempted to break it by whispering, nervously moving their legs, touching their hands, glancing across the circle, blinking their eyes. The climate they created was a watchful, controlled waiting, and only the more daring spoke up, saying they did not understand the meaning of this experience.

> **From a group's resistance to a working through of emotions (part 1)**
>
> Rosaria: I don't understand the purpose of this.
> Francesca: Yes, you explained, but I don't understand the point.
> Marco: We already have supervision from Clinical Reasoning.
> *They seem to fear the group's judgement and the conductor's judgement, and are afraid of exposing themselves.*
> Grace: There's resistance in the group; no one is speaking for fear of exposing themselves. Group supervision is different – you prepare your case, what you want to say.
> Pasqualina: In the group where I work, there is one team member who presents a case. It's different from here . . .
> *They find it difficult to speak out, to voice their thoughts.*
> Rosaria: You can cut the tension with a knife, feel the communication problem . . .
> Pasqualina: We have asked questions, you have answered, but we hear what we want to hear, half of the things don't . . .
> *The group differences begin to emerge – alliances, rivalries, difficulties, subgroups, sometimes in marked opposition like a battle. The students are surprised and alarmed by this.*

> *Previously they could avoid or deny uncomfortable feelings. Here they need to face them.*
> **Silvana:** We're not one united group but many groups.
> **Edda:** In 3 years I have initiated relationships but there are still some people that I am afraid to talk to. I worry that they might say to me 'Shut up, little girl.' I try to live calmly, otherwise I would cut my wrists . . .

The first stories they told related to institutions that accepted the students in fieldwork placements, and the whole group took a defensive attitude, underlining the deficiencies, the inefficiency, the staff hurriedness, the inadequate care for the patients, the lack of respect for other trainees. The university was accused of keeping theory and fieldwork divided, of not taking their inexperience into account, of being an insane university that sends them to places where they do not know what occupational therapy is, where they can learn nothing, etc.

The first scenic representation played out resulted in a kind of small riot, with interruptions from the circle and attempts to correct known situations. The conductor, from the beginning, took a firm stance because the rules of the setting had to be respected; she also used her reverie function and listens, containing the group by voicing their emotional nuances. This transition from primitive emotion to meaning and thinking requires growth at multiple levels. During the year, the group slowly changed, their attitudes became calmer; the conductor found that students were already sitting in a circle on her arrival, confidently waiting. With time the setting acquired a feeling of trust, a space where it was possible to voice and share difficulties and link them to different mental states.

The students' stories about therapy situations began to change, and through the dramas and work the group slowly came to understand the emotional states of each one of them. They no longer attacked the school, institutions or inadequate placements, but instead thought and talked of emotions, difficult moments with patients, dealing with the loss of limbs, minds, physical pain, their own anguish and defences put up to avoid the identifications, where they remain blocked and inert. The students were attempting to reach the correct distance with their patients through respectful listening together with the proposal of significant activities. They were learning to accommodate difficult communications and give patients hope for new possibilities in life.

From a group's resistance to a working through of emotions (part 2)

Tea: Seven weeks of training, many questions to ask. A 20-year-old boy falls from the 4th floor, there is nothing that helps the emotional aspects. There is only training, functional recovery. The psychologist was on holiday. How can you leave a boy like that . . . leave him there for a month?!

Marco: It's like that everywhere . . . speed . . . indifference . . . Thank goodness that you were there . . . with collage you helped . . . the collage activity helped.

Caty: With the collage the patient was able to speak of the satanic cults he was linked with, what he went through before jumping . . . and through playing out the scene we saw how the patient was relieved when he chose to cut up the images and could finally speak about himself.

Playing out the scene provides reflectivity and empathy, because it faces emotional truth without censorship. Observing, through acting the parts, how each of them faced their own difficulties and how this helps, encourages, promotes exchange and aids communication. In the group you can speak or remain silent, but this experience also compels those who would like to just sit on the sidelines to take an active part and become the protagonist of the scene acted out.

Silvia: It is important to face things that occurred during training. Seeing how others reacted helps.

Cosimo: But playing the scene scares me and makes me wonder why I have to act it out, here, in public, with all eyes upon me, what I did with the patient, my mistakes, no . . . why?

Cosimo was invited to play the part of an Alzheimer's patient, disorientated and abandoned in an establishment described by the students as a 'car park', where patients were physically restrained.

Cosimo: It was my first time . . . I had never felt what a patient feels! I felt anxiety . . . even now I feel sick . . . Now I understand . . . yes, I understand.

Lavinia recounts and acts out the evaluation with an autistic girl where the patient left the room to mix colours in the painting workshop, indifferent to the insistent demands of Lavinia, who called her back to the occupational therapy room.

Lavinia: In playing the scene it struck me that we trainees try to fill the silences – for me this is reassuring, for patients it is disturbing.

Maria: I have never heard of this, Lavinia. I'm sceptical, I don't understand its use.

Lavinia: I think differently. I have taken part and it has changed me. It's embarrassing, I almost fainted, but I've been through it and learnt. It was very helpful; experiencing the situation is different. I was very upset but I understood that I had overwhelmed the patient. Playing the scene helped me. It is an opportunity that we have. It is an opportunity!

Valeria: It's true. I struggled, in the beginning it bothered me, I didn't understand. Now, having acted out some situations, it's helped me.

Throughout the year the MOVI goal of coming closer to one's own emotions has taken shape slowly but progressively.

Rosaria: Before we spoke about problems to do with the school, now it's different . . .

Pasqualina: The silence . . . starting the morning with psychodrama, to start with our problems were unbearable! Now it's changed . . . now I feel differently. The silence no longer scares me; the silence is when we think.

Each student is able to discover the complexity of mental events, the richness of emotion.

Irina: This work moves me emotionally, while it answers my questions. I come out of the sessions richer, emptied but satisfied.

Grace: There should be more meetings; it should start in the second year.

Valeria: In these meetings there is a great team spirit. Now I let myself get involved, I like it and I feel the others more.

Each student had the impression of being more capable of understanding what was happening inside themselves through what had happened to others in the group and with the patients. Group communication improved, and group interaction was deepened thanks to a kind of mirroring: being seen by and seeing the others, they were able to know and accept hidden aspects of themselves that emerged within the group situation. It had a direct impact on their defensive narcissism, which had given way when they recognised in the others things that were also part of themselves.

Grace: We are all more secure, the roles don't scare us anymore, we can speak about ourselves to the others, and there is reflection on the part of all of us . . .

There is a sense of belonging that facilitates the continuation of the course. In fact, during collateral experiences in activity groups (e.g. in woodworking and cooking laboratories, the creation of personal books, etc.), the students show a greater ability to be together, to work together, to share experiences, to listen, to give space to the shy or more inhibited members. It helps them consider different groups in occupational therapy, with patients of all ages and with different pathologies. We propose that this experience is a voyage of discovery and self-insight that has promoted an ability to put the rational in touch with the emotional in each of them, as well as in the group as a whole.

Conclusions

During a training process, students should become better able to 'learn from the experience' of what happens in occupational therapy practice rooms. This means being in touch with one's internal world, immersing oneself in emotional states that pervade the encounter of humans with materials and objects, and an ability to move quickly between one and the other in a continuous and rapid movement.

Bion stated that the sense of reality for the individual has the same importance as food, water, air and waste elimination. Just as eating, drinking, or breathing inadequately can lead to harmful consequences in life, not making use of emotional experience produces disastrous effects on the development of personality (Bion, 1962).

'Learning from experience' requires a slow and profound reflection on the knowledge and questioning of our defensive shields that can prevent us from reaching an emotional truth – a therapeutic truth. A new look allows us to move closer to the pain in another's life in our role as rehabilitators, without being overcome by it, and in this way creating a complete transformation of the way we exercise our profession. This way of using feelings creates a closeness in the group; a solidarity in the frailness which is part of all of us; an awareness of sufferers' need to have professionals beside them who are capable of feeling and managing their deep projective identifications. This is what permits a real transmission of thought and emotion from one person to another. It is as if the products of the mind, created by images, emotions, bodily states, sensations, and the use of the real materials in our rooms (both those with form and those without), create the complex interwoven components in the therapeutic relationship.

Through the formative experience of case discussions using analytical psychodrama, students were able to get closer to their emotions, recognise them and be less afraid. This awareness of their own subjectivity has enriched and changed them, giving them a new significant starting point for their future profession.

Learning from baby observation

In fifteenth-century Tuscany, many well-known artists painted the breastfeeding Madonna, and still later even Leonardo da Vinci painted such scenes of mother and infant. My research, driven by a strong curiosity, took me to various places in Tuscany between Arezzo and Florence, where in simple votive chapels or small churches I found such 'Madonna del latte' frescoes on the central wall. These had an unusually strong emotional impact on me. They are simple paintings, by local artists, and often commissioned by women to express a feeling of gratitude for their prayers having been answered, or to appeal that their profound desire of fertility or breast milk be granted. The chapels are in areas where the limestone in the rivers nearby left white traces on the ground that looked like milk! With a mixture of ingenuousness and religious belief, childless women or mothers unable to breastfeed drank this water and immersed themselves completely in it, believing that, with the help of a Madonna, their prayers would be answered.

These ancient stories of the universal feelings of women and mothers, images that were depicted in soft colours, show us all how important it is for a mother to breastfeed her child and maintain the link that is broken by birth itself. Much has been written about this process of separation between mother and child, who are initially so close that they seem to share the same body. Winnicott (1971) wrote: 'Psychologically the infant takes from a breast that is part of the infant, and the mother gives milk to an infant that is part of herself' (p. 16).

Much has also been written about the nature of the bond created when a mother breastfeeds her newborn infant. It is considered a cornerstone of their future interactions that will influence all the relational processes that are to follow (Quagliata, 2002). It is as if the flow of milk were able to condense the sensory–emotional complexity of the mother and child and as if this were the central element around which the newborn might construct his or her mental state and early life.

This process can be seen during the baby observation experience introduced in England by Ester Bick, a Polish psychoanalyst, in 1948. It was an experience recognised as a precious instrument for studying the primitive (early) communication of the baby, and for helping the observers to develop their capacities for understanding and reflecting upon their own emotions (Bick, 1964), similar to the concepts of containment and reverie mentioned earlier in this chapter.

We have included the 'baby observation' in our Psychoanalytical Occupational Therapy training course, which has recently become a postgraduate Master's, 'Modello Vivaio in Occupational Therapy'. It is a course reserved for graduates in occupational therapy who want to explore further the emotional and relational concepts (from a psychoanalytic point of view) that are developed between patient, therapist and activity in the therapeutic process.

The observation process that we use follows the method introduced by Ester Bick in the UK Tavistock Clinic, and refers to an observation of a mother and her baby in their home. The objective recording of the data observed is intermixed with a description of the observer's own emotional resonance.

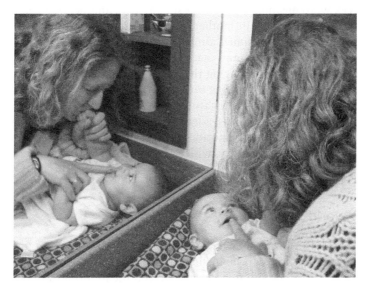

Figure 12.2 A mother speaks to her baby.

This very meaningful experience in the training process lasts for a year, with an observation at the baby's home once a week and a seminar group discussion every 15 days. Through the observation (without any attempt to intervene), the students learn to witness and to participate through silent listening in the complex and unique birth of a relationship. The experience constitutes a precious training in learning how to watch, to take in the details of what is happening and to pay attention to the sequences of actions and reactions. They learn the difficult task of coping with emotions in order to create the kind of distance necessary for welcoming, containing and supporting meaningful situations. Being able to watch without intervening is one of the most precious tools for a therapist, especially in our profession where 'doing' carries the risk of covering up (denying) and sometimes burying deep emotions.

Martha Harris, in a 1982 seminar, underlined the fact that to become a receptive observer, one needs to abstain from acting, and she put the emphasis on learning to watch, through the experience of the observation. She suggested watching and going back to things until the things themselves begin to talk (Harris, 1982). This learning is what happens during the observations and the free association to the material in the seminar groups.

Observing a newborn baby with its mother allows the student to be with both of them in their natural environment, together with the rest of the family. Father, brothers and sisters, grandparents and others are present while the two of them, mother and baby, search each other out, come together, put each other off. It is in this subtle and dynamic exchange that they create and develop their own particular relationship.

Observing is a little like filming them, as they live their lives through the range of infinite subtle happenings which are real, mental and emotional, and which give shape and character to their interaction. It is like witnessing and living time in slow motion, from week to week. For Dina Vallino (Vallino and Macciò, 2004) it is *kairos*, a Greek word meaning the time for staying with another. It is a slow time, to stay with a newborn child and its mother, to watch, to feel, to explore with eyes and mind their exchanges, sometimes almost imperceptible, which from the very beginning start their encounter and mark its future path.

It is a slow time for accompanying the newborn baby in its process of growth and change. It is a time for reflecting on the close connection between emotional and mental development, and the nature of the exchanges which represent the foundation of the baby's primitive identity. The quality of the exchanges can determine primitive bodily and emotional states in the newborn baby and leave subtle traces of precocious memory, which can affect the child and adult in future relationships.

The 'inner world'

The 'inner world' is a mysterious term, bringing to mind a deep sea; the part you cannot see on the surface, dark and silent, but densely populated, alive – a space which becomes animated with the appearance and the motions of the internalised personages.

Bion (1962) proposed that at the beginning of life there is no inner world, no theatre, no mind, no thoughts. There might be protothoughts, preconceptions, more surely a mix of sensations and emotions, mostly chaotic and tumultuous, without any natural place ready to receive them, digest them and transform them. It is similar to what happens when food is swallowed and the stomach keeps it, digests it and transforms it into nutrients for the body. An inner space is created for the digestion and the elaboration of emotions and sensations; it is formed gradually and is subject to numerous vicissitudes.

The inner world and the inner space were central concepts in the work of Klein and of Bion. For both, the relationship between the nursing baby and the breast was taken as a model for human relationships and for future development. For Klein (1946) it was through the processes of projection and introjection that the baby was able to create; for Bion (1962) it was through the model of container and contained that pre-thought could be transformed into thought.

The model of how thinking develops was introduced by Bion in 1962 in his well-known book *Learning from Experience*. It was to Klein's original theory that Bion added the idea of experience which precedes thought, a kind of mental state in which the mother possesses an intuitive knowledge of her baby's emotions, taking them into herself and trying to understand their meaning. This maternal function permits not only the containment of those states of anguish and suffering which the baby cannot hold in, called 'beta elements' by Bion (1962), but their transformation into 'alpha elements', which can be used for growing and thinking. The mother's mental function, which Bion calls 'reverie', is a sort of empathy through which the mother serves as a container for the baby's frustration. She receives and gives the first form to what is contained: that is, she is able to process her baby's primitive communication. She transforms his bodily sensations and chaotic and painful emotions into something that can have a meaning. This quality in the mother transmits to the baby the sensation of having a space in her mind, of being understood by her. Thanks to this empathic quality, a kind of internal story plot begins slowly to take form in the infants, expanding, consolidating, becoming with time their inner space where one day they will be able to elaborate the contents by themselves.

This process forms a kind of story plot, a fabric of connective tissue, keeping together all of the elements which go to form the inner world of a human being. This nascent self is trusted, and according to Klein (1952, 1957), is due to the introjection of an object which loves and protects the self and is loved and protected by a self. It is an object that Klein identifies with the breast, capable of giving nutriment with milk, with the mother's capable mind of thoughts. The breast becomes the original font of our internal world as well as a foundation for our future relationships with real figures from a real world. But the necessary condition for verifying the introjection of the good internal object, the good breast, is linked to the early containment experience discussed by Bion (1962), which is the capacity for 'reverie' (thoughtfulness) by the mother. (These concepts are discussed in more detail in Chapter 3.)

A mother who cannot provide this internal space offers a defective containing function, which from the start of life undermines the baby's search for adaptation with the mother. The failure of the maternal function of containment compromises the trustworthiness and the goodness of the object that the child introjects. These unfavourable conditions could interfere with the development of the baby's mental structure and with its capacity to metabolise the contents: in other words, interfere with the development of their inner world. This could lead to negative consequences such as the loss of imagination, of vitality, of the capacity for thought, for learning, for doing and for playing.

In our occupational therapy rooms we often treat patients with disturbances that seem to derive from the failure of the containment function and from the introjection of a persecutory internal object, a carrier of conflict. The emotions and the anguish which cannot be projected into a space that is able to receive them, tend to create confused, distorted, under-developed or even absent forms of attachment with the object. What predominates is a form of unhealthy dependence which makes the patients seem blocked at stages of development which do not allow either emotional or mental growth.

Occupational therapy considers 'doing' the central aspect of human experience and uses 'doing' as the focus of every therapeutic process. The psychoanalytic frame of reference introduces the affective dimension to the process of doing. As a result, the doing and playing, which make up every session of occupational therapy, take on representational (i.e. symbolic) and dynamic characteristics in the relationship between patient and therapist. The emotional movement, which is always present, fills the entire experience with communicative and transference significance. The therapists do and play together with the patients and gather and keep in their minds meanings and emotions during the rich succession of small things which happen in their interactions. A similar thing happens for the newborn baby when the mother's mind calms and digests the baby's shattering emotions so that they can be assimilated, and in this way she protects the baby from the difficult operation of transforming sensations into thoughts. For the patient, it is the therapist who contains the raw material, sometimes shattering, with her mind but also with her hands, and helps the patient to transform it. In time it will become material with form and meaning, and eventually the patient will be able to transform it as far as possible for themselves.

The following case example discusses the patient and the experience of the occupational therapist, and links the rich clinical material with the theory from infant observation.

Antonio

Antonio, an adolescent from a North African country, communicated his isolation, his closure, his apathy, his creeping depression. He had been referred from the public health service with a diagnosis of psychosis with autistic traits in addition to a conspicuous developmental delay. He was 13 years old and his internal world was 'a sort of cemetery' (Polacco, 1981, p. 309). Bion wrote that at the beginning thought is born from the temporary absence of the object, through the attempt to keep it alive in the mind. But Antonio had felt absence and loss too many times and for too long, and maybe it was because of this that he gave up. He had attacked his inner object, and had forgotten it. Gianna Polacco (1987) wrote: 'It is possible that one of the motives for a return to a two dimensionality is the defensive collapse of the internal space perceived as a receptacle for painful feelings and for frightening tenants that must be evacuated' (p. 105).

At the beginning in the therapy room Antonio did not look around him; he was not curious – he sat as if cowering perched on a stool. He seemed to withdraw into emptiness without giving any sign of response to what I was saying. I showed him the room and all of the things that he could use, but it seemed that nothing interested him; he was without energy, far away, and often bent his chin down to his chest, sticking out a long tongue that he pulled right back in closing his lips tightly and making strange movements with his mouth. He seemed to console himself, and he made me think of Marco, a 5-month-old infant who, when his mother returned to work, stayed for a long time during the observation with his small mouth in perpetual movement, sucking his tongue and his lips, as if he were looking after his need to be held together, to be contained, all by himself.

I felt that I had to try to keep Antonio together in a profound interaction with me, and at the same time give him a gradually growing sense of his own existence and reality. I needed to keep in mind the newborn's two great organizational principles which Alvarez (1992) described: 'a self that perceives, feels and thinks in relation to the object that perceives, feels and thinks' (p. 105).

I had started making up little games with my hands and his. He liked it when I took his hand and moved my fingers on the palm of his hand while I sang, 'In a piazza there's a crazy hen . . . pio . . . pio . . . pio.' He laughed and started to look at me. I sang other nursery rhymes and then wrote them in his personal story book which I took out in every session, starting a ritual that would give him a sense of stability and security. He was very interested in his body, face, feet, hands and hair, as if he were discovering them for the first time. Often he looked in the mirror and explored himself, sticking out his long tongue, laughing and looking, almost surprised. He often showed me that his hands were white inside and he invited me to put my hands in his.

When he discovered the container of glass frames used for making slides, he was amazed when we put one of his hairs between two pieces of glass and he could see it greatly enlarged, projected on to the white wall.

He often took off his shoes, and when I had him stand on a piece of paper to be able to draw around it, he seemed struck by having so much of my attention. He took on the task of cutting out the footprints and pasting them into his personal story book. After that we did the same with his hands and then added a playful self-portrait drawn in a simple way with eyes, nose, mouth and a tuft of hair. Before drawing them he had checked the presence and the form of each feature of his face at the mirror, touching them lightly with his fingers.

At the beginning of each session, he leafed through his personal story book, stopping at the foot- and handprints and his portrait. He would touch them delicately, then look at me smiling, as if by seeing himself reflected in my eyes he had confirmation of his existence. It seemed to me that Antonio was beginning to get to know his body as if he were recovering or constructing a bodily self that could integrate and organise itself in his inner space. Slowly he started to look around, to touch some of the materials in the room, to open drawers, to look in his box, on which he even succeeded in writing his name with a big blue marker.

Many times Antonio had brought feelings of suffering and abandonment to our work together. He had shown himself as empty and apathetic, and many times I had tried to contain his suffering, helping him to understand it. But I had also tried to form a bridge over the empty spaces between him and me with body games, simple materials and his personal story book, in an attempt to help him leave a trace of himself, of his existence, of his reality. Having a space in my mind and being understood by me were the conditions that permitted him to develop a space in his own mind, and gradually, step by step, a sense of action, of intentionality, of reciprocity, of thought, which permitted him to leave a mark on his world.

In our work with patients having severe psychotic or autistic pathologies, there are often situations that remind us about our observation of the newborn baby and mother. Having this experience is helpful in managing the inevitable therapeutic difficulties that arise in clinical work. Some of these patients seem to live in purely motor and sensory territories, without any apparent access to the mind, perhaps even lacking an apparatus for thinking. Being in contact with them means starting from points of attraction that are in harmony with a primitive sensory use centred on auditory, tactile, olfactory experiences, which remind us of the first months in the life of an infant with his or her own mother. She acts as a container that holds and gives a first form to the contained, which means to the primitive communications of her baby, transforming his bodily sensations and his chaotic emotions into something that can have meaning. Therapists, as seen in the following example, can offer the same opportunity for transferring unbearable emotion into action and thought.

Pietro

Pietro takes hold of a plastic container with two eggs inside . . . the eggs fall on the floor. Pietro, indifferent to the eggs, crushes the hard plastic between his fingers and brings it to his mouth with a sinister crackling sound. Then in his zigzagging way he goes away from me and then comes back again while I am picking up the eggs, which I put in a bowl. Pietro looks at me, then looks at the yolks which are still whole in the bowl. 'Those are yolks, egg yolks,' I tell him. 'We can use them for making a little cake, or some dough-nuts, or . . . who knows', and I look at him with an expression between amused and questioning. This makes me think of the baby observation of Nicola, in which his mother Sonia places herself in the path of her 4-month-old baby's glance, which is directed at the coffee that is percolating in a transparent moka coffee pot, gurgling and emitting a delicious fragrance. She comments to the baby, 'You like coffee . . . right? Who knows when you will be able to drink it! But I'll give you a taste if you want.' The baby agitates his hands and gurgles and cries out happily while he watches his mother, who continues to talk to him.

Pietro does almost the same thing when he unexpectedly cries out, looks at me with laughing eyes, beats on his chest with a hand and keeps sucking the plastic container, but stays close to me and does not go to take refuge in the corner of the room.

Exactly as it is for a mother and her infant, containment, synchrony, empathy and reciprocity constitute the fundamental elements of the relationship between therapist and patient.

Conclusions

Mattie Harris (1987), like Bick, saw infant observation as a training tool. She begins by explaining the value of learning how to observe. This is reinforced by Miller (2008), who wrote:

> The aim of the Baby Observation is two-fold. First the student gains highly privileged and detailed access to processes whereby a child grows up emotionally, socially and intellectually within a family. Secondly, the student is enabled to develop the capacity to observe, and to observe in a rich and tonal sense. Watching and listening, developing an eye and an ear for detail and power subsequently to record it, must be allied to the highest possible degree of emotional receptivity.
>
> (pp. 40–41)

The students in the Vivaio Master's programme prepare a clinical paper at the end of the course on their experiences with the baby observation. This brings together what they learn from the observation itself and how this has influenced their professional practice. One student described it as 'Being there for taking in and listening, for being close, with attention, following step by step the path that the other travels, without the haste that used to drive me.' Another student wrote: 'I feel stronger and more able to contain my own emotions and therefore I can contain those of my patients as well.'

Although the awareness of emotions gives meaning and depth to the rehabilitative function of our profession and enriches the field of its application, occupational therapy has not developed space in its busy training curriculum to having direct knowledge of this emotional world of baby and mother.

The introduction of baby observation into our training had the objective of permitting the participants to approach and recognise emotional states, understand their meaning and slowly assimilate the ways and the means to render these states tolerable in order to be able to use them as occasions for facilitating growth in every occupational therapy process.

Afterword

The experiences of psychodrama and infant observation facilitate the students' discovery and knowledge of each other, enabling them better to *be* together and work together.

Particular attention is needed regarding the emotional aspects that arise, persist and change in the dynamics between therapist, patient and activities. We would urge every school of occupational therapy to create special training modules which will help students to recognise emotions and create more profitable relationships in their therapeutic encounters.

References

Alvarez, A. (1992) *Il compagno vivo*. Rome: Astrolabio.

Anzieu, D. (1956) *Le psychodrame analitique chez l'enfant et l'adolescent*. Paris: Presses Universitaires de France, 1979.

Bick, E. (1964) Notes on infant observation in psychoanalytic training. *International Journal of Psycho-Analysis*, 45, 558–566.

Bion, W. R. (1961) *Experiences in Groups and Other Papers*. Hove: Brunner.

Bion, W. R. (1962) *Learning from Experience*. London: Heinemann.

Breuer, J., and Freud, S. (1892-1895) *Studies on Hysteria: Case Histories*. London: Penguin.

Brook, P. (1995) *The Open Door*. New York: Theatre Communications Group, Inc., 2001.

Ferenczi, T. (1921) *Further Contributions to the Theory and Technique of Psycho-analysis*. London: Karnac, 1994.

Freud, S. (1909) *Five Lectures on Psycho-analysis*. Oxford: Oxford University Press, 1999.

Freud, S. (1911) The handling of dream-interpretation in psycho-analysis. In The Standard Edition of the Complete Psychological Works of Sigmund Freud (Vol. XII, pp. 89–96): The Case of Schreber, Papers on Technique and Other Works. London: Hogarth Press, 2000.

Freud, S. (1912) Recommendations to physicians practising psycho-analysis. In *The Standard Edition of the Complete Psychological Works of Sigmund Freud* (Vol. X.I.I. pp. 109–120): *The Case of Schreber, Papers on Technique and Other Works*. London: Hogarth Press, 1999.

Harris, M. (1982) Personal notes during a seminar with Martha Harris and Donald Meltzer on the Infant Observation in Rome.

Harris, M. (1987) Contribution of observation of mother–infant interaction and development to the equipment of a psychoanalyst or psychoanalytic psychotherapist. In *Collected Papers of Martha Harris and Esther Bick* (pp. 225–239). Perthshire: Clunie Press.

Kaes, R. (1972) *Le psychodrame psychanalitique de groupe*. Paris: Dunod, 1999.

Klein, M. (1929) Personification in the play of children. In *Love, Guilt and Reparation and Other Works: The Writings of Melanie Klein* (Vol. 1)London: Hogarth Press, 1975.

Klein, M. (1946) Notes on some schizoid mechanisms. In *Love, Guilt and Reparation and Other Works: The Writings of Melanie Klein* (Vol. 1)London: Hogarth Press, 1975.

Klein, M. (1952) Some theoretical conclusions regarding the emotional life of the infant. In *Envy and Gratitude and Other Works: The Writings of Melanie Klein* (Vol. 2)London: Hogarth Press, 1975.

Klein, M. (1957) Envy and gratitude. In *Envy and Gratitude and Other Works: The Writings of Melanie Klein* (Vol. 2)London: Hogarth Press, 1975.

Lebovici, S. (1974) A combination of psychodrama and group psychotherapy. In S.De Schill (ed.), *The Challenge for Group Psychotherapy*. New York: International Universities Press.

Lemoine, P., and Lemoine, G. (1973) *Lo psicodramma*. Milan: Feltrinelli.

Marineau, R. F. (1989) *Levy Moreno 1889-1974: Father of Psychodrama, Sociometry, and Group Psychotherapy*. London and New York: Tavistock and Routledge.

Miglietta, D. (1998) *I sentimenti in scena*. Turin: Utet Libreria Università.

Miglietta, D., and Pani, R. (2006) *Dal teatro allo Psicodramma analitico*. Milan: Franco Angeli.

Miller, L. (2008) *The relation of infant observation to clinical practice in an under-fives counselling service*. In *'What Can the Matter Be?' Therapeutic Interventions with Parents, Infants and Young Children* (pp. 38–53). London: Karnac.

Polacco, H. G. (1981) La doppia deprivazione. In M. Boston and D. Daws (eds), *Il lavoro psicoterapico con bambini e adolescenti*. Naples: Liguori.

Polacco, H. G. (1987) *Psychotherapy with Several Deprived Children*. London: Routledge and Kegan Paul.

Quagliata, E. (ed.) (2002) *Un bisogno vitale*. Rome: Astrolabio, 2007.

Vallino, D., and Macciò, M. (2004) *Essere neonati*. Rome: Borla.

Winnicott, D. W. (1971) *Playing and Reality*. London: Routledge.

13 The Relational Space of Supervision

Margaret Daniel

The aim of this chapter is to reintroduce psychodynamic thinking as part of occupational therapy's core skills to enhance the profession's identity through a process of critical reflection. It also aims to reawaken the core relationship skills for occupational therapists who use themselves as therapeutic agents in their work. By addressing the less conscious aspects of this relational work, I will examine how the 'felt experience' of the emotional material can impact on the therapist. I will also describe how occupational therapists can utilise this type of experience to enhance and inform their practice.

Dundas (1990), in his work on the use of sand play, suggested that if people can get in touch with their creative process, 'they find the road opens to lead them out of their difficulties' (p. 5). This chapter explores whether occupational therapists can use a supervisory space to explore their creative potential, as it may open up richness to their therapeutic work.

Introduction

Some of the features of a psychodynamic approach remain valuable to current occupational therapy within clinical practice and supervision by bringing 'feelings' back into the relationship. In this chapter I would like to invite readers to begin to think about how their clinical practice and supervision could be enhanced through a psychodynamic perspective that can add to our professional reasoning as occupational therapists. What I mean is that Occupational Therapists are open and able to work in areas of emotional pain and can often be invited to react. It is important to recognise that feelings will be evoked in the clinician, and rather than viewing this as a sign of weakness, practitioners need to think of it as informing part of their everyday work.

The psychotherapist Patrick Casement (2002) described the idea of an inter-relational space for clinical supervision, which he believed involved learning

Psychoanalytic Thinking in Occupational Therapy: Symbolic, Relational and Transformative, First Edition.
Lindsey Nicholls, Julie Cunningham Piergrossi, Carolina de Sena Gibertoni and Margaret A. Daniel.
© 2013 John Wiley & Sons, Ltd. Published 2013 by John Wiley & Sons, Ltd.

together even from what we might perceive as our mistakes, as we all have areas that are out of our awareness. How the activity unfolds can reveal areas that have gone unnoticed in the space that is created, both in therapy and in supervision.

The traditional role of supervision in occupational therapy

Supervision can be an elusive process to define and within the profession of occupational therapy it has been described by the College of Occupational Therapists (COT) as 'a professional relationship which ensures good standards of practice and encourages professional development' (1990, p. 1). The criteria were extended in 1997 to incorporate governance and accountability issues, and as the occupational therapy educators, Gaitskell and Morley (2008) note in their opinion piece, the occupational therapy profession is eager to sanction supervision as a legal and professional requirement (College of Occupational Therapists, 2005, 2006; Department of Health, 2004). However, this is without a clear understanding as to its application, evidence base and level of competency.

Influenced by the papers written by Hunter and Blair (1999) and Sweeney, Webley and Teacher (2001a, 2001b, 2001c), a small survey of newly qualified occupational therapists (Gaitskell and Morley, 2008) highlighted concerns that there continues to be confusion over the task of supervision. Their findings note a lack of solid training in supervision and affirm that the supervisory role is often professionally acquired, which may not take into account the craftsmanship of the supervisory skills. Geraldine Shipton (2000) trained as an occupational therapist and went on to become a psychotherapist and trainer. She would endorse the idea that a more in-depth training is required to explore the complexity of supervision that is not profession specific.

The continuing confusion as to whether clinical supervision needs to separate the combined role of supervisor, as manager and clinician, remains an ongoing debate (see also Kleiser and Cox, 2008). Although the roles overlap, managerial supervision essentially has the interests of the organisation in mind, whereas clinical supervision sets out to enhance the clinician's effectiveness. If managerially driven, clinical supervision could become an appraisal tool that monitors fitness to practise, losing site of the non-hierarchical supportive culture that clinical supervision can offer therapists in fulfilling their everyday tasks. The educators and clinicians, Hughes and Pengelly (1998) would advise caution if clinical supervision is being used as a form of 'quality control', as the unsettled environment of constant change can induce primitive ways of operating. Lynch, Hancox and Happell (2008), from a nursing perspective, believe that clinical supervision requires clear delineation from line management supervision. They point out that, although line managers and the organisation are involved in setting up the process of clinical supervision, 'they have no role within the supervisory relationship itself' (p. 11). From the occupational therapy literature reviewed, many of the authors (Frye, 1990; Finlay, 2002; Kleiser and Cox, 2008; Mackenzie and Beecraft, 2004) recommend or consider a clinical form of supervision to be essential, yet this seems to be an area that has had limited study.

If we look back to the 1960s, Fidler and Fidler (1963, p. 250) believed that supervision provided a 'learning and growing' experience that expanded self-awareness through gaining a better understanding of others. This awareness was an essential part of organisational and departmental functioning. The process of supervision had further depth, which lay in its collaborative approach and led to greater understanding. They saw that the sharing of material, in a creative way, helped to raise morale and intensify cohesiveness.

Fidler and Fidler's (1963) theoretical model was derived from other professional groups (e.g. social workers) who were informed by psychoanalytic ideas, and the Fidlers regarded this approach as readily transferable to occupational therapy practice and supervision. Almost 50 years later, this method would still seem to be in keeping with the profession's current ethos. As Smyth and Joice (2011) highlight, there is a growing need for appropriate and accessible supervision for mental health occupational therapists, who currently contribute to the psychological therapies and require multi-layered levels of intervention within their practice. I believe that clinical supervision, from a supportive and relational perspective, has the potential to add a richer dimension to the supervisory process by developing an enquiring interest into the affective process (Daniel and Blair, 2002). Within our current climate of financial constraints, this form of professional supervision may not be easily accessible or relevant to everyone. It will take creativity to negotiate and to identify clinicians who use a psychodynamic approach, and who may be in a position to mentor or supervise clinical work in addition to a line-managed approach.

The psychodynamic influence to supervision

From a psychodynamic perspective Jacobs, David and Meyer (1995) combine to describe supervision as 'a process during which supervisor and supervisee are learning together – about the patient, about one another, and about themselves' (p. 6). They also note that the process of supervision will vary depending on the supervisory couple's level of experience and the supervisor's approach. Underpinning the structure and purpose of supervision is a theoretical model, which like a metaphorical coat hanger helps to form and give order to the clinical material. The model that is interwoven throughout this chapter is a relational model, which offers a containing and reliable framework from which to explore the range of issues brought to supervision.

Frawley-O'Dea and Sarnat (2001) describe three aspects relevant to a relational model of supervision, which are used to address the basic supervisory task. They suggest that consideration should be given to the level of the supervisor's power, which can range from a didactic factual stance, through to a supportive companionable position, where power is acknowledged and used by the supervisor to remain open and curious to the process. The second aspect focuses on the supervisor paying attention to the therapeutic relationship and the supervisory relationship and the influence these relationships have on the organisation itself. The final aspect views the supervisor as more than a teacher or a curious questioner who holds and contains the feelings which arise. Indeed, Frawley-O'Dea and Sarnat (2001) point out that the supervisor is also required to monitor his or her own physical and emotional part in the process.

As the occupational therapy educator Boaz (2003) mentions, the craft of supervision within health and social care stems from psychoanalytic ideas. Sigmund Freud's (1856–1939) writings on the subject are sparse, but his weekly meetings with interested colleagues, where cases were presented and techniques discussed, became the nursery ground from which the concept of supervised practice emerged (Jacobs, David and Meyer, 1995).

In contrast to Freud's rather distant and detached manner, his associate and friend, Sándor Ferenczi (1873–1933), had a warmer and more engaging approach. He was interested in the relationship and how the therapeutic work impacted on the therapist, where, insightfully, he considered that some of the techniques used in psychoanalysis could themselves trigger an emotional reaction (Ferenczi, 1933). Ferenczi's supervisee, Michael Balint, extended his ideas by recognising how the power imbalance in relationships could be utilised through negotiation and where issues could be shared. He considered that a more educative style could constrain and control, resulting in a loss of independent thinking (Frawley-O'Dea and Sarnat, 2001).

It is interesting to note that similar issues regarding the dual role of supervisor, as manager and clinician, were being discussed within the psychoanalytic world as early as the 1920s. Within psychoanalysis, a split was created between the two schools of thinking. One school of thought (Viennese) felt that the tasks of teacher and therapist needed to be separated into different individual roles, whereas the other school of thought (Hungarian) preferred an integrative approach (Carroll, 1996).

Within our day-to-day working environment, the distressing stories we hear from our clients can have the capacity to render us helpless. The intensity of the feelings can hamper our ability to listen, and remain motivated and engaged, as the enormity of the feelings can overwhelm us. In addition, we have to keep in mind that our internal and external environments influence how we hear and think about our work (Heard, Lake and McCluskey, 2009; Heard, McCluskey and Lake, 2011). We bring all our past encounters to the supervisory space and can easily be influenced by a remark, a look or a gesture that echoes past moments when we felt ridiculed, shamed, stupid or exposed (Encke, 2008). These disquieting thoughts may be triggered in the supervisory space by something that reminds us of a previous time. If we can be aware that these conscious thoughts from the past exist, we can open up the experience by managing our fluctuating feelings so that we can remain curious to what the feelings may be conveying (Heard, Lake and McCluskey, 2009; Heard, McCluskey and Lake, 2011). Supervision that is informed by psychoanalytic concepts can add a richer dimension that helps us to move beyond our experiences and into a further realm of possibility.

The landscape of possibility

From his longstanding work within therapeutic communities, the psychoanalyst Robert Hinshelwood (2001) regards clinical supervision as offering a thinking container, which functions as a way of absorbing the clinicians' emotional needs, stirred up from the nature of their working environment. By helping to make sense of what is happening in the ward or community, regarding interpersonal dynamics, a broader perspective can be gained from what is being mirrored by the whole department on behalf of the organisation or particular individual splits on behalf of the team, such as scapegoating. Just as a mother helps her child to understand the felt experience, so the supervisor assists the supervisee to identify the emotional landscape that has been formed by the external environment, without infantilising the supervisee (Hawkins and Shohet, 1989).

To achieve effective supervision, Donald Schön (1987) described how practitioners required space to think about their practice by either 'reflecting-on-action' (in order to recollect past events) or 'reflecting-in-action' (to be able to maintain an ability to think alongside the situation). Essential to this, Wilfred Bion (1975), as a psychoanalyst and group consultant, believed the practitioner had to be able to tolerate the uncertainty of what is not yet within our awareness. Harold Searles (1955) and Janet Mattinson (1975) took an adventurous step in extending this further, to include what was happening in the actual supervisory relationship. They illustrate how the material brought to supervision could be responded to, in gleaning further understanding of the therapeutic relationship, which Hughes and Pengelly (1998) believe is a micro-representation of the organisation itself.

Similarly, as Julie Cunningham Piergrossi describes in Chapter 4, the British psychoanalyst Donald Winnicott (1971) used the concept of 'transitional space' to influence the social scientist Harold Bridger's (1978) thinking about organisational change. Bridger believed that learning through experience was dual purpose. It requires the clinician to get the work done. Bion (1961) describes this as the 'primary task' but it also requires a point of 'review', in which to examine how the real task has been undertaken. The supervisor has the potential to create a space for the supervisee to think about and reflect on how the work is affecting them, as well as how they, themselves, are affecting the clinical work around them. If an enabling atmosphere of support and understanding can be engendered with a mutual space to explore and contemplate the supervisee's role, a deeper understanding can be gained through this containing environment (Hinshelwood, 2001; Heard, Lake and McCluskey, 2009; Heard, McCluskey and Lake, 2011). The supervisor also has to keep the supervisory dyad in context. To take account of the bigger picture of the organisation itself, as a way of attending to the emotional health and well-being of staff and to maximise their potential and enhance best practice (Driscoll, 2000). Winnicott (1971) ascribes to the most creative expression of learning, which he believes happens through play. In adults the process of play absorbs our interests and culturally leads to new discoveries that Heard, Lake and McCluskey (2009, p. 8) call 'Eureka' moments, which serve to validate and enrich the supervisory process.

Paying attention to the 'doing'

An experienced occupational therapist came to supervision with some pictures that a 22-year-old woman with an eating disorder had painted. From the start of the supervisory session the pair were absorbed in the visual material and excited by forming ideas as to how this activity could be developed.

The supervisor was monitoring the therapist's behaviour and began to realise that they were possibly caught up in enacting something from the therapy session itself (parallel process). The supervisor drew attention to what was happening to them and wondered if there was anything about their behaviour and feelings that was familiar to the supervisee.

The supervisee recalled how he had been 'lit up' by the woman's work and excitedly drawn to helping her come up with more ideas that she could develop. They began to think about what their actions and feelings were, setting them in context and considering whether their heightened activity was communicating something from the person herself.

The supervisor realised that he had been out of his usual pattern and he too had been drawn to focusing on the artwork within the session, wanting to offer ideas as to how the paintings could be developed. He realised that he had lost sight of the person behind the work. Here was a young lady who had difficulty eating and perhaps one way that she dealt with her condition was to distract others from seeing her problem.

In the supervisory session, both the supervisor and supervisee could recognise that they were 'hungry' to come up with ideas and that the therapy session too had been 'filled up' with ideas that the occupational therapist rather frantically wanted her to 'digest'. The defensive activity being enacted needed to be understood. The energy and excitement within both the therapy and supervision sessions had to be managed in a way that did not overwhelm and that could be returned in a more digestible way to the person.

Reflective practice

Reflective practice has gained attention in the NHS as a valuable tool for maintaining continuing professional development (Healthcare Professional Council, 2005; Department of Health, 2004). It can be understood as learning from experience and can be separate from supervision. Hughes and Pengelly (1998) note that there is a tendency to use the term loosely, in giving thoughtful consideration or feeding back about what has been happening previously. Spalding (1998) also considers that occupational therapy has split the concept of reflective practice into positive and negative, so that outcomes can be improved: for example, what went well or not so well, and how it could be improved. From an occupational therapy background and with further training as a psychoanalytic psychotherapist, Robertson (2001) would contest that this attempt to manage uncertainty in supervision can lose its creative and non-judgemental qualities.

One way in which Wylie and Rooney (2006) suggest this can be addressed for novice occupational therapists is through the valuable asset of peer supervision. Peer supervision is a learning space that can help to build confidence and skills, in a supportive and reflective way. The authors suggest that this can assist new therapists to manage their anxiety level, as they do not wish to be seen as incompetent. Moore (2012), however, emphasises Casement's (2002) view that practitioners need to learn from situations that do not always go to plan and should be able to review alternative actions without creating a culture of blame.

To be reflective the therapist has to have a capacity to take in the outer information, to ponder on the process and consider alternative possibilities. As a reflective practitioner, Schön (1991) suggests we require the felt hunch of intuition that can be considered in context to the event and to the bigger organisational picture. By using our internal experience, which Casement (1985, p. 29) calls the 'internal supervisor', insight can also be gained: for instance, producing an idea that has hitherto been hidden. It could be a way to resolve a difficulty or gain a glimpse of personal insight.

The supervisory space

The supervisory space is an active area with features that resemble Winnicott's (1971) concept of 'holding'; having a safe and consistent environment, which can facilitate 'good enough' supervision (p. 10). This object relations perspective recognises that supervision is not about making the work perfect. It requires an area with boundaries that is consistent, uninterrupted and active, with space to think (play) about the live material as it is presented (Hawkins and Shohet, 1998). Sweeney, Webley and Teacher (2001c, p. 430) attribute Winnicott's notion of the 'good enough mother' to Hawkins and Shohet (1989), and through the analogy emphasise the importance for supervisors themselves of addressing the emotional impact that this role has on them.

Winnicott would consider that we have to develop a 'capacity to be alone' (1971, p. 47), containing material on behalf of the people we work with (transference), which is held in mind and brought to supervision. It can then be discussed in a way that gives room to explore the inner emotions evoked by the experience (projection). The supervisor attempts to translate the projections, active on the boundary of the supervisee's work, having the ability to give an impression of what is happening in order to hold, or contain, the raw emotional material that has been absorbed from the ongoing work. This gives an opportunity to explore the organisational as well as the clinical perspective, which may offer a further dimension to the process (Frawley-O'Dea and Sarnat, 2001).

Working in the field of trauma, Jochen Encke (2008) draws on the passion of supervision, believing that it is more than simply a space to reflect. He beautifully illustrates the vitality of the creative process: 'When supervision provides a space in which stories and problems are seen as the gateway to a new dimension of reality, rather than merely as issues which need solving, for me at that moment it becomes passionate supervision' (p. 20).

Within the supervisory space, the partnership has the ability to examine the story in a more relaxed and thought-provoking way, which loosens the gaze to uncover what is beyond the material brought to supervision. It works something like the magic eye books (Burder, 1994) that get people staring for hours, trying to pick out the undiscovered image which lies hidden beyond the dots. The knack is to relax your gaze and, as your eyes adjust, a three-dimensional scene unfolds, sweeping past the coloured dots and exposing a landscape not seen at first glance. We can apply this idea to supervision, where the work presented and the reflection of the event or issue may cover up what lies beyond the selected material. If the supervisory couple can extend their gaze beyond the concrete story, a landscape of possibility may yield new and creative ways of thinking together about the work (Encke, 2008).

The way in which supervision is performed gives the supervisee a psychological skin and a boundary to their practice, resembling the psychoanalyst Anzieu's (1999) concept of a 'psychic skin' (p. 324). To act as a protective shield, the skin requires a porous quality so that the emotional content of the work can be felt without overwhelming. As with the work, supervision, like consultancy, can fluctuate between thinking and feeling. Within the space the supervisor can 'pull back' so as to think about the supervision process and similarly 'open up' to the felt experience in the larger organisation outside. In context, the narrative may also reflect the politics of the changing organisation and its setting in contemporary society: for example, the staff may be tolerating inadequate resources as they put up with/have got used to normalising deprivation, a feature of their clinical work alongside a reflection of the organisation. What can then happen is a response to anxiety and helplessness in an inability to influence the situation (Hughes and Pengelly, 1998).

Supervision can inspire through recognising and owning the projections that empower as well as assist in unravelling the everyday felt experiences. This space has the potential for creativity, which, Winnicott (1971) believed, involved the inclusion of imaginative play alongside reality. However, from an art therapist's perspective, Jennings (1983) would contest that it requires the courage to step beyond the frame of what is known with the addition of determination and dedication. At this boundary of change, anxiety is heightened, as the transition from known to unknown is fraught with risk and pain. Out of this absence or loss of the object that went before, symbols evolve and new resources can become accessible.

At the core of subjectivity are an individual's deliberate choices and intentions, which form the basis of their emerging identity (Heard, Lake and McCluskey, 2009; Heard, McCluskey and Lake, 2011). Without this, there can be no emotional development, and as Duncan (1999, p. 521) contests, the profession of occupational therapy has to have developmentally reached its 'adolescent identity crisis' before it can be sufficiently mature to have confidence in the professional repertoire that defines its role within the cultural landscape of mental health. There is the possibility for a psychodynamic attitude to enhance practice through accessing the inner emotional life, which can offer a more balanced overview of the dynamics of an individual's actions – an enabling place, such as clinical supervision, which can replenish a supervisee's energy, contain and soothe his or her anxiety and fear, as well as providing room to be curious and creative (Heard, Lake and McCluskey, 2009; Heard, McCluskey and Lake, 2011).

The focus of emotions within the supervisory relationship has for many years been overlooked in occupational therapy, and the impact of feelings aroused in the therapist has often been considered inappropriate to acknowledge, unless psychodynamically trained. The occupational therapist Gita Ingram (2001) would consider that psychodynamic ideas provide occupational therapists, who are involved in human relations, with a greater understanding of their practice and that the method mitres well with a holistic approach. Ingram notes that supervision is a developing relationship that is not part of a 'fire-fighting' response to a crisis and emphasises the need to create a supportive external environment where the live material can be brought for discussion. The supervisory space defines a physical and emotional structure that gives time to meaningfully think about what is being presented in both verbal and non-verbal ways. It seems to me that clinical supervision needs to incorporate a playful quality, similar to a dance in which the supervisory couple glide through the work into an effortless place. To achieve this, the supervisor partners the therapist, and they discover the pace, steps and rhythm that they require, which will inevitably lead to points where supervisory toes are trodden on as the couple learn the steps together.

Considering boundaries in supervision

The idea of seeing therapy as having a boundary was described by Marion Milner (1950) in what she calls the 'frame'. Milner trained in psychotherapy and had an interest in art. She described how, like a picture, the therapeutic setting required a boundary that could define what was inside and what was outside. As sleep provides the frame for dreams (Milner, 1987), so the therapeutic activity is framed within the setting, which includes a space to create, with time and the uniformity of the therapist's behaviour. In that way, trust can be built to explore and think symbolically about emotions, fears and the deeper relationship of the individual and/or the group. The outer frame can be defined by the structure of the room and offers containment, while within there is an inner frame that is less tangible and constructed in the contract of the work to be done together.

A further way of establishing a clear boundary within supervision is through establishing a contract at the start of the process, in which the task and remit of the work are jointly agreed. This will set up a climate of transparency, which can give clarity to what the supervisor and supervisee both want from the experience and expect of each other. These basic building blocks to supervision are also open to review and reshaping as the supervisory relationship develops (Hughes and Pengelly, 1997).

It can be likened to being part of the audience in a play: the supervisor has to watch and listen to the individuality of the story as it unfolds. As the supervisee relates the felt experience, the supervisor is attuning to the narrative from both a physical and an emotional position. The supervisor's felt experience can be used to enhance and inform the therapeutic journey, which will have been built on through the supervisor's own experience of being supervised. A symbolic space is available to the supervisor, to think creatively about the experience that the unfolding picture offers as a glimpse into the therapeutic relationship (Frawley-O'Dea and Sarnat, 2001).

Enlightening the supervisory process: the means by which the client is brought to supervision

The American psychoanalyst Harold Searles (1955) used the term 'reflection process', which is now recognised as 'parallel process'. According to Frawley-O'Dea and Sarnat (2001, p. 173), parallel process can be defined as 'the means by which key relational patterns of one dyad come to influence the relational configuration of the other dyad'. Material that the therapist has unconsciously linked onto can be unwittingly brought from the therapy session into the supervisory space (and vice versa). The material is then enacted within supervision. The supervisor, who is less involved, may be able to catch the supervisory interaction, to elicit whether their actions could be informing them about the person's inner environment. This is not always a matching process and can be subtle. It encourages exploration at different levels to uncover potential meaning that can enrich the work: for example, the therapist may be talking about how tired she felt when working with a lady who was depressed. Matching this in supervision may be the supervisor noticing that he has become extremely distracted and disinterested as he listens to the story. However, Searles (1955) adopts a cautionary tone when he suggests that this experience may be more about the supervisor's reaction (i.e. countertransference) to the supervisee than stemming from therapy itself.

More than 50 years ago the psychotherapist Paula Heimann (1950, 1960) described the concept of countertransference and how essential it was for a therapist to have an awareness of how their inner mood and outward actions could be influenced by their ability to attune to the person's unconscious. Sandler, Dare and Holder (1973) introduce countertransference as a generalised term for the therapist's emotions, shaped by the unconscious material offered by the person and possibly containing both helpful and pathological elements. However, if this term is made over-inclusive, Fonagy and Target (2003) believe it can lead to confusion in locating the source of the evoked emotions. Heimann (1950) considered that it added valuable material from the unprocessed thoughts and intolerable emotions that were hard to acknowledge and own.

Taking this idea further, Searles (1955) believed that what became stirred up between the person and the therapist could also be replicated (i.e. parallel process) in the supervisory encounter. He shifted the focus onto the supervisory relationship where the supervisor and supervisee take into account what was happening between them in the 'live' relationship. It also took account of unfinished work, which may have been brought unconsciously into the supervisory space. I consider this a valuable way in which occupational therapy can utilise the inner resources that are accessible if the therapist listens to their own emotional world and monitors their altering activity. However, Sandler, Dare and Holder (1973) warn that if the therapist becomes over-reliant on their intuition, the person's material may get ignored.

At the Spring Sutherland Trust Lecture in 2009, the psychotherapist Jane Polden (2010) described her supervisory work within the prison service, where the staff and inmates could be drawn into the more physiological state of mirroring or imitating those around them. She drew on the work of Italian neuroscientist Rizzolatti who helped discovered mirror neurones (Rizzolatti, Fadigo, Gallese and Fogassi, 1996). His research shows that by observing someone's actions, similar areas in the brain become activated: for example, a monkey watching another monkey pick up and eat a banana will have fired up the same motor area in the brain concerned with carrying out the task, even when the monkey is not directly involved.

We can all examine this physiological reaction in ourselves when we think about how hard it is to stifle a yawn when someone else has been yawning; how difficult it is to keep your mouth closed when spoon feeding a baby; or how aroused we can become when supporting our football team just as they are about to score a goal. We are all unconsciously drawing on our primitive relational processes when we attune to the other in trying to understand what they might be feeling (McCluskey, 2010).

Central to the work of an occupational therapist is the 'doing process' of activity/occupation, and as Julie Cunningham Piergrossi illustrates in Chapter 7, the activity is an emotional communication process where symbols and choices can tell us more about someone's unconscious internal environment. The level of questioning enquiry we take will differ depending on our skills and supports. Gail Fidler (Fidler and Fidler, 1963) would encourage occupational therapists to acknowledge that feelings can be operationalised in doing and are signals to use as therapists. The following example illustrates a piece of work taken to supervision and the importance of having space to think and feel about what may lie behind the unfolding activity choice both for the person and for the therapist.

The gift

Alex is a 45-year-old man who came to therapy the day after the death of his wife (which is quite unusual), as there was concern that he might be suicidal. Although his wife's death was anticipated when it actually happened, he felt unprepared and due to the level of his distress he began attending occupational therapy in a psychotherapy day hospital. However hard he had prepared for his wife's ending, it still came as a shock. One of his wife's problems was sleep apnoea and at night he would keep the radio on to drown out the noise of her breathing. Yet at the same time he was also listening out, in case her breathing stopped.

Therapy took place over a 2-year period and we met on a weekly basis. After a period of settling, his favoured choice of activity was woodwork in which he could plane, hammer and sand lumps of wood. During the sessions his anger was close to the surface along side his acute distress. It became especially acute when he tried to say his wife's name, which he was unable to do. To manage this he would shift his focus on to the drainpipe on the adjacent building, and greet it, saying, 'Good morning, Mr Drainpipe', or check that the dead fly on the window ledge was still there. Throughout the sessions he would lace his comments with black humour, which made me feel I had to stay constantly alert, unable to let my thoughts drift for a moment. This heightened feeling of alertness left me feeling drained.

A pattern began to emerge in which he would count down the last 5 minutes of the session and, as he left, would struggle to open the door, trying to turn the handle or push instead of pull. One of the objects he constructed was a large robust wedge, which he presented to me at the end of the session as a gift to be used as a doorstop for the department, which I accepted.

As the ending of therapy approached, Alex was able to talk more about his wife without becoming overwhelmed. He began to talk about events leading up to her death. As on so many other occasions, she had become unwell but this time she had asked her husband not to leave her alone. His son was en route to their house and to speed up getting his wife to hospital he rushed out of the house to pick him up. He was away less than 5 minutes, but when he returned he found that his wife had slipped into a coma and she did not recover consciousness. His guilt in leaving her was enormous.

As we worked towards the ending of his sessions, Christmas was approaching. On his way out of the session prior to Christmas, he left a present on my desk, which I did not open until later. I discovered it was a beautiful silver bracelet. It was something I would wear but it left me feeling terrible, as if I were holding on to a secret. In supervision my supervisor asked me what I wanted to do. I would have loved to have kept the present but knew that it was not for me to accept.

At his third last session in the New Year, I met with him again and explained that he had given me a fantastic present but that I was unable to accept it, as it was an intimate gift for someone who was special. He became angry, saying that there was nothing to it. He stormed out of the room – with no problem negotiating the door this time – and took the present with him.

He cancelled his penultimate session and arrived at his final session saying, 'Well, I bet you were worried!' He went on to explain that his son had been taken unwell and he had to take him to hospital. He looked round the room, noting the drainpipe and the dead fly that had still not been cleared away. He had been thinking over the previous meeting and thought that what I had said made sense. He had kept his plan to himself and not spoken about it to his colleagues at work; in a way, he realised that was a sort of secret. He now considered that these sessions had been a rehearsal for the future – if he could survive my rejection of his gift and return to face me, then having a relationship again with someone else might be possible.

On reflection

There are many issues going on within this example, on both a conscious and an unconscious level. In having clinical supervision alongside this work, I was able to consider some of the different levels that had been presented. The relational gap between the therapist and the person bridges worlds between people. It is a paradox of union and separation. The gift of the handmade wedge maintained a symbolic connection to me as well as signifying an absence – a way of gradually becoming separate as therapy's ending became more apparent, as well as symbolising the idea of leaving the door open.

The second 'wedge' of the silver bracelet was different and had to be handed back. It was something that I felt was not for me, but it had to be understood for what it represented. Supervision gave me a space to examine how the work was impacting on me and what I was discovering about the relationship we had together.

The wedge for Alex was a way to redo the past; to keep the door open, be able to say goodbye to his wife and not leave – all the things he had wanted but been unable to do. Alex was repeating the 'wedge' (connection) with me and I needed to give it back (in the form of returning the bracelet). Supervision gave me a place in which to express my feelings of anxiety and apprehension; a way that helped contain my discomfort and awkwardness as I returned the bracelet, so that it did not spill further into the organisation through managerial and ethical issues. If I had kept the bracelet, I would have been caught up in the 'never-ending circle' which carried with it the space/gap contained in the heart of the bracelet. It was also the space/gap left by Alex's wife and with the added loss of myself as his therapist. In giving back the bracelet, I was helping him to make sense of his loss, by closing the circle and confirming that the space/gap could be contained.

Over these sessions I guess it felt like I had to give 100 per cent concentration all the time and I always felt tired having brought his case to supervision. In supervision I had the ability to explore my need to stay in heightened alertness, almost holding my breath. Supervision helped me to see that in reality it would not have been possible to continue with that level of attention, just as it had been unrealistic for Alex to listen constantly to his wife's breathing. If we were to continue to 'wedge' the sessions open, then Alex's time in therapy would never close. His sessions needed to end and I had to 'close' the circle, confirming perhaps that sometimes it is possible to leave someone without the other dying.

In being able to return for his last two sessions, Alex was able to express his anger at feeling rejected in the declining of the gift, but he also had the potential to consider what lay ahead. He was able to think in a different way and to do it in my presence. How do you stop, let go, without rejection? Like the personal and private experience of death itself, therapy has to end, leaving a gap and disappointment but at the same time new potential; another 'wedge' to be managed. Ending with me was important, and without the supervisory space in which to explore and contain my own anxieties, the work would have lost its deeper meaning. I leave you with the thought of what the 'wedge' would mean to you in your supervision?

Conclusions

Supervision has a multiplicity of styles and approaches. This chapter offers occupational therapists a relational way of thinking about the creative process of supervision by reintroducing psychodynamic concepts that acknowledge how our inner 'emotional' environment can inform our clinical practice. The theory, I suspect, needs to be put into context with the felt experience of clinical practice. For that reason, it is thinking about the live interaction in the therapeutic and supervisory relationship, and the wider organisation, that brings its potency to life. Through a clinical supervisory relationship, the creative process can be contained, reflected on and perhaps understood in a supportive, companionable way, offering an enlightening and revitalising perspective in which the activity choice and symbols can enrich the process.

References

Anzieu, D. (1999) The group ego-skin. *Group Analysis*, 32 (3), 319–330.
Bion, W.R. (1961) *Experiences in Groups*. London: Tavistock, 1968.
Bion, W. R. (1975) *A Memoir of the Future, Book One: The Dream*. London: Karnac 1990.
Boaz, M. (2003) Supervision in practice. *Therapy Weekly*, 11 September.
Bridger, H. (1978) The increasing relevance of group processes and changing values for understanding and coping with stress at work. In C. L. Cooper and R. Payne (eds), *Stress at Work*. Chichester: John Wiley & Sons, org.
Burder, D. (1994) *Super Stereogram*. London: Boxtree.
Carroll, M. (1996) *Counsellor Supervision: Theory, Skills and Practice*. London: Continuum.
Casement, P. (1985) *On Learning from the Patient*. London: Routledge.
Casement, P. (2002) *Learning From Our Mistakes: Beyond Dogma in Psychoanalysis and Psychotherapy*. Hove: Brunner Routledge.
College of Occupational Therapists (1990) *Statement on Supervision in Occupational Therapy*. London: College of Occupational Therapists.
College of Occupational Therapists (1997) *Statement on Supervision in Occupational Therapy*. London: College of Occupational Therapists.
College of Occupational Therapists (2005) *College of Occupational Therapists: Code of Ethics and Professional Conduct*. London: College of Occupational Therapists.
College of Occupational Therapists (2006) *Management Briefing: Supervision*. London: College of Occupational Therapists.
Daniel, M. A., and Blair, S. E. E. (2002) A psychodynamic approach to clinical supervision: 1. *British Journal of Therapy and Rehabilitation*, 9 (6), 237–240.
Department of Health (2004) *The Knowledge and Skills Framework and the Development Review Process*. London: Department of Health.
Driscoll, J. (2000) *Practising Clinical Supervision: A Reflective Approach*. Edinburgh: Royal College of Nursing, Bailliere Tindall.
Duncan, E. (1999) Occupational therapy in mental health: It is time to recognise that it has come of age. *British Journal of Occupational Therapy*, 62 (11), 521–522.
Dundas, E. T. (1990) *Symbols Come Alive in the Sand*. London: Coventure.
Encke, J. (2008) 'Breaking the box: Supervision – A challenge to free ourselves'. In R. Shohet (ed.), *Passionate Supervision*. London: Jessica Kingsley.

Ferenczi, S. (1933) Confusion of tongues. In J. M. Masson (ed.), *The Assault on Truth: Freud's Suppression of the Seduction Theory* (pp. 145–188) Harmondsworth: Penguin, 1984.

Fidler, G., and Fidler, J. (1963) *Occupational Therapy as a Communication Process in Psychiatry*. New York: Macmillan.

Finlay, L. (2002) Groupwork. In J. Creek (ed.), *Occupational Therapy and Mental Health* (pp. 245–264) Edinburgh: Churchill Livingstone.

Fonagy, P., and Target, M. (2003) *Psychoanalytic Theories: Perspectives from Developmental Psychopathology*. London: Whurr.

Frawley-O'Dea, M. G., and Sarnat, J. E. (2001) *The Supervisory Relationship: A Contemporary Psychodynamic Approach*. New York: Guilford Press.

Frye, B. (1990) Art and multiple personality disorder: An expressive framework for occupational therapy. *American Journal of Occupational Therapy*, 44 (11), 1013–1022.

Gaitskell, S., and Morley, M. (2008) Supervision in occupational therapy: How are we doing? *British Journal of Occupational Therapy*, 71 (3), 119–121.

Hawkins, P., and Shohet, R. (1989) *Supervision in the Helping Professions: An Individual, Group and Organisational Approach*. Milton Keynes: Open University Press.

Healthcare Professional Council (2005) *Continuing Professional Development: Key Decisions*. London: Healthcare Professional Council.

Heard, D., Lake, B., and McCluskey, U. (2009) *Attachment Therapy with Adolescents and Adults: Theory and Practice Post Bowlby*. London: Karnac.

Heard, D., McCluskey, U, and Lake, B. (2011) *Attachment Therapy with Adolescents and Adults: Theory and Practice Post Bowlby* (2nd edn) London: Karnac.

Heimann, P. (1950) On counter-transference. *International Journal of Psycho-Analysis*, 31, 81–84.

Heimann, P. (1960) Counter-transference. *British Journal of Medical Psychology*, 33, 9–15.

Hinshelwood, R. D. (2001) *Thinking about Institutions: Milieux and Madness*. London: Jessica Kingsley.

Hughes, L., and Pengelly, P. (1998) *Staff Supervision in a Turbulent Environment: Managing Process and Task in Front-Line Services* (2nd edn) London: Jessica Kingsley.

Hunter, E. P., and Blair, S. E. E. (1999) Staff supervision for occupational therapists. *British Journal of Occupational Therapy*, 62 (8), 344–350.

Ingram, G. (2001) Psychodynamic theories. In L. Lougher (ed.), *Occupational Therapy for Child and Adolescent Mental Health* (pp. 97–110) London: Churchill Livingstone.

Jacobs, D., David, P., and Meyer, D. (1995) *The Supervisory Encounter: A Guide for Teachers of Psychodynamic Psychotherapy and Psychoanalysis*. New Haven, CT: Yale University Press.

Jennings, S. (ed.) (1983) *Creative Therapy*. London: Kemple Press.

Kleiser, H., and Cox, D. L. (2008) The integration of clinical and managerial supervision: A critical literature review. *British Journal of Occupational Therapy*, 71 (1), 2–12.

Lynch, L., Hancox, K., and Happell, B. (2008) *Clinical Supervision for Nurses*. Chichester: Wiley-Blackwell.

Mackenzie, A., and Beecraft, S. (2004) The use of psychodynamic observation as a tool for learning and reflective practice when working with older adults. *British Journal of Occupational Therapy*, 67 (12), 533–539.

Mattinson, J. (1975) *The Reflection Process in Casework Supervision*. London: Tavistock.

McCluskey, U. (2010) Understanding the self and understanding therapy: An attachment perspective. *Context, February*, 29–32.

Milner, M. (1950) *On Not Being Able to Paint*. London: Heinemann.

Milner, M. (1987) *The Suppressed Madness of Sane Men*. London: Tavistock.

Moore, E. (2012) Patients with personality disorder: The impact on staff and the need for supervision. *Advances in Psychiatric Treatment*, 18 (1), 44–55.

Polden, J. (2010) Behind closed doors. *British Journal of Psychotherapy*, 26 (4), 502–521.

Rizzolatti, G., Fadigo, L., Gallese, V., and Fogassi, L. (1996) Premotor cortex and the recognition of motor actions. *Cognitive Brain Research*, 3, 131–41.

Robertson, J. (2001) Supervision and stress. *British Journal of Occupational Therapy*, 64 (10), 517.

Sandler, J., Dare, C., and Holder, A. (1973) *The Patient and the Analyst* (revised edn) London: Karnac, 1992.

Shohet, R. (2008) *Passionate Supervision*. London: Jessica Kingsley.

Schön, D. A. (1987) *The Reflective Practitioner: How Professionals Think in Action*. New York: Arena.

Schön, D.A. (1991) *The Reflective Turn: Case Studies In and Out of Educational Practice*. New York: Teachers Press.

Searles, H. (1955) The informational value of the supervisor's emotional experience. *In Collected Papers on Schizophrenia and Related Subjects* (pp. 157–76) London: Karnac, 1993.

Shipton, G. (2000) *Supervision of Psychotherapy and Counselling: Making a Place to Think*. Buckingham: Open University Press.

Smyth, G., and Joice, A. (2011) Psychological therapies in Scotland. *OTNews*, 19 (9), 29.

Spalding, N. (1998) Reflection in professional development: A personal experience. *British Journal of Therapy and Rehabilitation*, 5 (7), 379–382.

Sweeney, G., Webley, P., and Teacher, A. (2001a) Supervision in occupational therapy. Part 1: The supervisor's anxieties. *British Journal of Occupational Therapy*, 64 (7), 337–345.

Sweeney, G., Webley, P., and Teacher, A. (2001b) Supervision in occupational therapy. Part 2: The supervisee's dilemmas. *British Journal of Occupational Therapy*, 64 (8), 380–386.

Sweeney, G., Webley, P., and Teacher, A. (2001c) Supervision in occupational therapy. Part 3: Accommodating the supervisor and the supervisee. *British Journal of Occupational Therapy*, 64 (9), 426–431.

Winnicott, D. W. (1971) *Play and Reality*. London: Routledge.

Wylie, H., and Rooney, C. (2006) Peer supervision: A priceless experience. *OTNews, February*, 24.

Index

Psychoanalytic Thinking in Occupational Therapy: Symbolic, Relational and Transformative, First Edition.
Lindsey Nicholls, Julie Cunningham Piergrossi, Carolina de Sena Gibertoni and Margaret A. Daniel.
© 2013 John Wiley & Sons, Ltd. Published 2013 by John Wiley & Sons, Ltd.

Printed and bound by CPI Group (UK) Ltd, Croydon, CR0 4YY

27/10/2024

14580296-0003